Penguin Books

Penguin Nursing Revision Notes
GENERAL MEDICAL NURSING

Other titles in this series:

Penguin Nursing Revision Notes
Advisory Editor: P. A. Downie

■ General Medical Nursing

Revised edition

Penguin Books

PENGUIN BOOKS

Published by the Penguin Group
27 Wrights Lane, London W 8 5 T Z, England
Viking Penguin Inc., 40 West 23rd Street, New York, New York 10010, USA
Penguin Books Australia Ltd, Ringwood, Victoria, Australia
Penguin Books Canada Ltd, 2801 John Street, Markham, Ontario, Canada L 3 R 1 B 4
Penguin Books (N Z) Ltd, 182–190 Wairau Road, Auckland 10, New Zealand

Penguin Books Ltd, Registered Offices: Harmondsworth, Middlesex, England

First published 1982
This revised edition first published in Penguin Books 1989
10 9 8 7 6 5 4 3 2 1

Copyright © Penguin Books Ltd, 1982, 1989
All rights reserved

Made and printed in Great Britain by
Cox and Wyman Ltd, Reading, Berks.
Filmset in 9/10½ pt Linotron 202 Galliard by
Rowland Phototypesetting Ltd, Bury St Edmunds, Suffolk

Contents

Contents

Advisory editor's note

This series of revision aids first saw the light of day in the early 1980s and has been reprinted numerous times thus indicating that the books fulfil a real need. Now they have been revised and updated. Many nurses, both tutors and ward sisters, have helped and advised in these revisions; they are too numerous to list individually but the warm thanks of the publishers and the advisory editor are extended to each of them.

These small books are not textbooks, *but* revision aids; consequently they aim to indicate principles and outlines rather than in-depth descriptions. Where specific treatments and care are discussed the reader should remember that they are not necessarily the only methods. All hospitals have their own laid-down treatment procedures and protocols and nurses must always apprise themselves of these.

Clinical terminology has been used throughout, though where there is an anatomical or scientific term this is shown also, and both terms are used simultaneously.

Care plans are shown in some of the books, but all the books lay emphasis on the four parts of the nursing process which can be turned into effective care plans, namely assessment, planning, implementation and evaluation. *Care* for patients is the *raison d'être* of all nursing and while these books are essentially revision aids for examinations, they nevertheless emphasize the nurse's role in the direct care of the patient.

Examinations might be described as 'necessary evils' in that they provide a means of ensuring that a person has reached an acceptable standard of competence. These books are intended as aids to help attain this standard; essentially they are for learners rather than nurses undergoing post-basic courses. Suggestions to help both study and the actual examination are included as is a short list of relevant reading. Specific references have not been included but learners are advised to make full use of their School of Nursing library and to seek help in learning how to seek out references from the librarian and their tutors.

In the 1850s, Florence Nightingale discussing how to teach nurses to nurse wrote in her *Notes on Nursing*, 'I do not pretend to teach her how, I ask her to teach herself, and for this purpose I venture to give her some hints.' Now, some hundred years on it falls to Penguin Books Limited to offer 'some hints' to the learner nurse of the present day as she prepares for her examinations.

P.D.
Norwich, 1988

Introduction

Patients are admitted to a medical ward for many different reasons and for varying lengths of time. Generally, the patients do not require surgery and do not expect to have an operation in the sense that a patient would if he were admitted to a surgical ward. The management of the patient is likely to involve monitoring the patient's condition and response to therapy, tests, investigations, drug therapy, diets, and so on. This is not to say that medical nursing does not involve an understanding of the principles of surgery, as a patient receiving medical treatment may well require a general anaesthetic and have to be prepared for theatre for certain investigations.

A patient may be admitted to the medical ward from the waiting list having had knowledge of the impending admission for some time, or as an emergency without any preparation for admission. Although both categories of patient are admitted to a medical ward, their needs may be entirely different and partly dictated by the type of admission.

When two patients are admitted with the same disease process, they may not require the same help and support while in hospital. Even if the problems they both experience are the same (which may or may not be directly related to their medical condition) they may require different nursing intervention to help overcome the problem. The nurse must understand that the patient, like herself, is an *individual*, a member of a family and a member of society; trying to isolate the patient from this is failing to see the *whole* patient. Unfortunately, if the patient is not seen as an *individual* in this way, it is possible for him to come into hospital, be treated for the particular disease and go home, without his needs having been met or even recognized. Some patients may have so many problems that only some of their needs can be met, but the nurse should have the ability to recognize that a patient may have certain needs because of, or in spite of, the disease process for which he or she is being treated. This can be achieved only by careful and continuous assessment of the patient as a whole.

When the patient comes into hospital it is all too easy to see the patient only in that setting and to forget how traumatic an experience it is for the family and the total disruption this hospitalization may cause, even if it is only for a brief period when considered in terms of life span. Decisions may now have to be made by another member of the family, who may feel inadequate to do so; financial difficulties may arise for the people visiting;

emotional difficulties may arise out of the separation which is caused by illness, and the practicalities of maintaining a daily routine may be put under severe strain. These problems may be made easier or more difficult by other factors, e.g. the family's ability to cope with this kind of pressure, the progress that their relative is making in hospital, the length of stay and the patient's attitude towards his illness. However, when all concerned – the family, the patient and those caring for the patient – are aware of the difficulties and have an understanding attitude, these will go a long way to support the patient and his family.

The nurse must have a knowledge of the diagnosis and the disease processes for which the patient has been admitted to hospital, but she must also realize that the patient may not be so much concerned with the disease pathology as with the effect that it has on his daily living activities, and on his family. This will be influenced by the patient's ability to understand his illness and its implications, his ability to ask questions, to talk about and explain how he feels. It is because patients have different perceptions and fears about their illnesses that they ask so many different questions about the effect the illness will have on them. This is because their way of life, their work, their hobbies, their indulgence in sporting activities may be affected in the long term.

1 General principles of medical nursing

The *general* principles of medical nursing are considered so that the learner can use them as a source of reference when applying them to the care of each patient.

■ ADMISSION

■ Planned

a From the waiting list.
b From another ward/hospital where specific treatment has commenced.

■ Emergency

a From home or work via the GP or emergency services (sudden event).
b Via the GP or consultant domiciliary visit following a period of illness at home.
c Via the outpatient clinic.
d Transfer from another ward/hospital where patient was being treated for the same or different condition.

■ Reasons for admission

a The patient requires treatment which has to be carried out under continuous medical supervision.
b The patient has an acute condition which requires prompt medical intervention.
c To assess the extent of a disease.
d For investigations to determine a medical diagnosis.
e For terminal care.

■ MEDICAL HISTORY AND PHYSICAL EXAMINATION

All patients admitted to a medical ward will undergo a full physical examination and have a careful history taken by the doctor. The patient's condition and type of admission will decide the treatment and investigations which will follow. Some of the investigations ordered by the doctor will be routine while others will be specific; the doctor may also ask the nursing staff to carry out specific observations of the patient at regular intervals. The nurse should be familiar with what is routine, have a basic understanding of the specific investigations that may be required, and of the nurse's responsibilities in relation to these investigations. Note will also be made of the drugs the patient may be taking; any drugs that the patient brings with him into hospital should be dealt with according to hospital policy. The doctor will prescribe the drugs that the patient requires while in hospital, which may or may not be the same as those which he was taking prior to the admission. Often at this point the doctor explains to the patient any treatment and investigations which may be necessary.

■ PSYCHOLOGICAL FACTORS

Admission to hospital can be a very distressing experience for a patient. To be able to listen to patients and give them the opportunity to talk about their fears and anxieties is an important part of the nurse's function. She should also be able to refer patients when necessary to people who are better able to help them cope with their problems. Maintaining good communication with patients and their families and keeping them informed of all relevant information at all times is also important.

Much fear and anxiety can be relieved at the time of admission if the patient and his family are made to feel welcome. Following this initial meeting the relatives ought to be able to go home with ease of mind, knowing that the patient will be cared for by people who are concerned for him as a person.

■ NUTRITION

The nurse should be able to assess the nutritional state of the patient and to report her observations to the medical staff. It may be that the patient is in a state of poor nutrition for many different reasons. It may be directly related to the disease process, or to other factors – psychological or socioeconomic. The patient may require a special diet as part of the treatment for his condition, e.g. a reduction or an increase in calories, or a reduction or increase in the protein in the diet; vitamin supplements may also be necessary.

Occasionally it may be necessary to restore a patient to a good nutritional state by intravenous feeding. Any fluid and electrolyte imbalance may also be corrected in the same way. The doctor will set up the infusion and it is the nurse's responsibility to ensure it is in working order and that the fluid regime prescribed is maintained and recorded. For certain investigations there may be times when oral food and fluids will be withheld from the patient for a specified period of time, and the necessity for this should be explained to the patient.

■ ELIMINATION

■ Bowels

The patient may be receiving specific drug treatment for disease of the bowel which must be administered as instructed by the doctor. It is important to establish with each patient his usual pattern of elimination. The nurse should recognize the need for privacy, the provision of facilities for handwashing following the use of the bedpan/commode/sanichair, and the importance of observing the stool, both its colour and consistency, and to report any abnormalities. It may be necessary to obtain specimens of stool for specific laboratory investigations. The nurse should also appreciate the importance of the prevention of constipation.

■ Bladder

All patients admitted to a medical ward will have their urine tested routinely. All urine should be observed for its colour and volume. Urine may also have to be obtained for specific laboratory investigations. It is important for the nurse to follow specific laboratory instructions for the collection of various specimens. The importance of accurately measuring and recording urinary output for patients with certain medical conditions cannot be over-emphasized.

■ SKIN AND HYGIENE

On admission and throughout his stay in hospital, observation should be made of the patient's skin colour, texture and cleanliness. The nurse should assess the patient's ability to perform his own personal hygiene and this will range from the patient's being able to care for himself without assistance, through the varying degrees of assistance, to total dependency.

The aim should be to keep the patient's skin clean and intact. Careful drying of the skin will help prevent soreness in those areas of the body that sweat.

Special care of the skin will be required when the patient is pyrexial, with frequent washes when the patient is feeling 'hot and sweaty', frequent changes of clothing and use of cotton bed linen and nightwear, which are cooler for the patient. The patient's hair should be observed, kept clean and in good condition, the nails cleaned and manicured. It may be necessary to ask the chiropodist to undertake care for the feet and toenails.

■ BREATHING

Patients with breathing difficulties due to specific diseases may well be in a medical ward; such cases will be dealt with later in the text. In any case the ward should be well ventilated and patients discouraged from smoking. The doctor may ask the nurses to carry out specific observations of a patient's respiratory rate, volume and character along with other observations that may be necessary. Specific chest physiotherapy may be ordered and specimens of the patient's sputum may be required. It is sometimes necessary to measure the amount of sputum produced and to observe its colour. Oxygen therapy may be required and will be prescribed by the doctor; the nurse must ensure the safety and comfort of the patient during its administration.

■ MOBILIZATION

The nurse should be able to assess the degree of mobility of each patient and to decide what measures may be taken to help a patient with decreased mobility. Some patients will need to have their positions in bed changed by the nurse, other patients given suitable aids (if their condition permits) may be able to help with lifts, others may be able to move themselves in bed. The degree of mobility will help the nurse to select the appropriate aids to be used to help prevent the breakdown of the patient's skin. It must be stressed that equipment used to prevent the development of pressure sores is not a substitute for vigilant observation, nursing care and the continuous change of position for the relief of pressure.

The position in which the patient is nursed is either that in which he is most comfortable, or a position dictated by the medical condition. It is for the nurse to ensure that whichever position, he is safe and comfortable.

■ OBSERVATIONS

The observations which a nurse may be asked to carry out will be those general observations of the patient's appearance together with specific observations such as:
a Temperature.
b Pulse (rate, rhythm, volume).
c Respirations (rate, depth, character).
d Blood pressure.
e Level of consciousness and response of patient.
Other observations may have to be made depending on the patient's condition and any doctor's instructions such as 'supine and standing' blood pressure.

The frequency with which these observations are recorded is decided by the patient's condition, his progress or otherwise in response to therapy.

■ ADMINISTRATION OF DRUGS

This section will be particularly useful to learners who will shortly be attempting the ward-based practical assessment of the administration of drugs. Specific rules and regulations governing these practical assessments may vary from one training school to another, but the following general principles will serve as a useful guide.

1 You should familiarize yourself with the examination's policy in your particular training school.

2 You should be aware of your right to appeal in the event of a referral or fail and how to follow this procedure.

3 You should inform the ward sister of the pending assessment so that maximum guidance can be given.

4 You must be familiar with the local drugs' policy and be able to state the importance of adhering to it.

5 You should be able to identify routes by which drugs can be administered.

6 It is expected that the learner will be safe to administer drugs by following the correct procedure for identifying the patient, and that the correct drug and dosage is given at the prescribed time by the route instructed on the prescription sheet, and the administration correctly recorded.

7 You should be able to state the action of common drugs and those which you are administering.

8 You should be able to state the importance of recognizing any side-effects of the drugs.

9 You should be able to explain the procedure governing the storage and administration of controlled drugs as currently practised in your training school.

10 You should be able to clear away equipment and utensils used and to complete the procedure correctly according to hospital policy.

■ INVESTIGATIONS

Most of the common investigations will be mentioned in due course in relation to specific conditions. The following principles may be applied to most of the investigatory procedures.

■ Preparation

The doctor will explain to the patient what the investigation entails. The nurse may have to explain to the patient that it is necessary to refrain from eating and drinking for a period of time, or that a certain area of the body needs to be shaved, and so on. Equipment may have to be obtained and prepared. Certain observations may have to be performed prior to a procedure and occasionally a consent form may have to be completed and signed by the patient. This is obtained by the doctor. Other hospital departments may have to be informed of the investigation, and the correct specimen containers may have to be obtained. The doctor may prescribe a sedative and it is the nurse's responsibility to see that it is administered at the appropriate time.

■ During the procedure

When it is necessary, the nurse should ensure that the patient assumes the correct position for the procedure. Throughout the course of the procedure the nurse should remain with the patient, observing and reassuring the patient. It may be necessary for the nurse to accompany the patient to another department for the investigation. The doctor may require assistance with some procedures and where this is necessary it is appropriate for two nurses to be available, one to assist the doctor, and one to be with the patient. The nurse must always show the doctor concerned the containers, with their labels, of any drugs that may be administered during the course of the procedure, *before* the drug is administered. The nurse should ensure that any specimens obtained are placed in the correct containers and sent to the laboratory, labelled and accompanied by the appropriate form or forms.

■ **Following the procedure**

The patient should be observed for any untoward effects. The nurse should ensure that the patient is nursed in the appropriate position; any necessary instructions should be clearly explained to the patient, e.g. he may be advised not to get up for a certain period of time. The doctor may, if it is possible, indicate to the patient how long it will take for the result of the investigation to be obtained. Equipment should be cleaned and where appropriate, safely and correctly disposed of. The nurse should report immediately to the medical staff any abnormalities in relation to observations made, or any complaints the patient makes.

■ NURSING REPORTS

Nurses are required to record the nursing care administered to every patient in the Kardex or the nursing care plans, and progress notes may be appropriate. Writing should be legible and reports brief and accurate; but they should not be brief to the exclusion of important detail and only abbreviations *approved* in relation to drug dosage should be used. Should an error be made during the course of writing, the nurse should simply put a line through it, initial the error and write it out correctly. Signatures rather than initials should be used on completion, and the progress notes should reflect the aims of the nursing care planned for the patient.

■ REHABILITATION

The rehabilitation that patients require varies considerably. Each patient should be assessed at the outset and continuously in relation to the amount and type of help and advice they may require before their discharge home. Other disciplines, such as occupational therapist, physiotherapist, speech therapist, medical social worker, resettlement officer, will almost certainly need to be consulted to achieve full rehabilitation within the particular patient's limitations.

2 The heart and blood vessels

The objectives of this section are:
1 To outline the relevant anatomy and physiology.
2 To identify common diseases of the heart and blood vessels.
3 To describe the total management of the patient undergoing investigations and treatment of conditions identified.

■ THE HEART (Fig. 1)

The heart is a hollow muscular organ situated in the mediastinum. It is centrally placed tilting slightly to the left. It has an apex and a base. The heart receives its blood supply via the coronary arteries and is drained by veins which include the coronary sinus.

The heart is divided into four chambers, two on the right and two on the left side (the atria and ventricles). Normally there is no contact between the right and left sides which are separated by the septum. The layers of the heart are arranged from the inside as follows:

Endocardium: smooth squamous epithelium.

Myocardium: cardiac muscle (special properties of conduction and rhythmicity).

Pericardium: a serous membrane which encloses the heart and great vessels. It has an outer fibrous coat and a double inner serous coat which is adherent to the heart and the inner surface of the outer layer; the 'space' between the 2 inner layers is filled with fluid.

The unidirectional flow of blood through the heart is achieved by the presence of the atrioventricular (AV) and semilunar valves:

□ *Right side*
Atrioventricular valve (tricuspid).
Semilunar valve (pulmonary valve) → pulmonary artery.

□ *Left side*
Atrioventricular valve (mitral valve).
Semilunar valve (aortic valve) → aorta.

Occasionally valves are damaged and become incompetent or stenosed.

■ Function of the heart

Oxygenated blood leaves the lungs and enters the left atrium of the heart through the pumonary veins, passes through the mitral valve into the left ventricle, from where it is pumped via the aorta around the body, returning to the right atrium of the heart, depleted in oxygen, through the superior and inferior vena cavae. From the right atrium the blood passes through the tricuspid valve into the right ventricle, from where it is pumped to the lungs, via the pulmonary artery, picking up oxygen and releasing carbon dioxide before returning to its left atrium through the pulmonary veins.

The heart continuously pumps blood around the body. The amount of blood pumped out by each ventricle every minute is 5 litres, this is termed the cardiac output. The total volume of blood in the body is about 5 litres, which means, therefore, that the blood circulates the body once every minute. The heart beats at approximately 70 beats a minute and this is called the heart rate. It is the heart rate that the nurse is measuring when she takes the pulse.

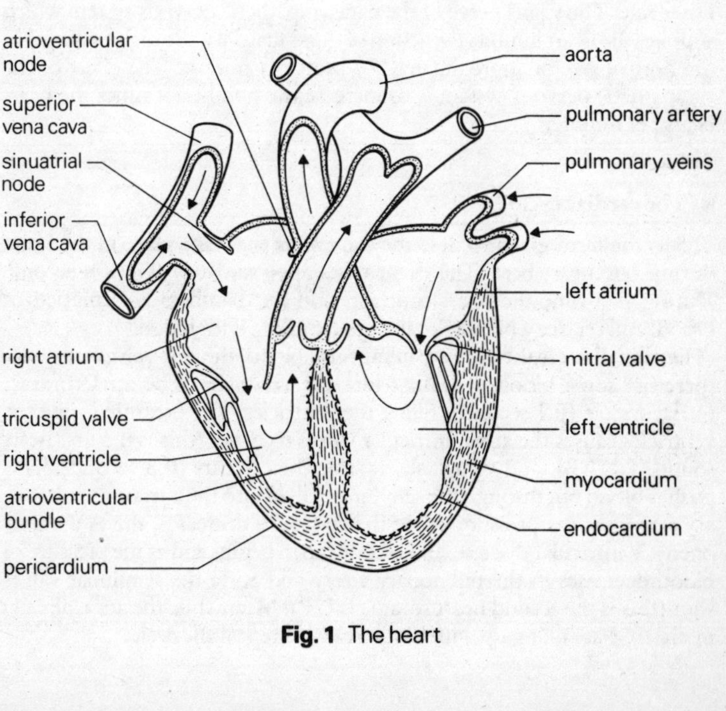

Fig. 1 The heart

■ The conducting mechanism of the heart

This consists of:

a Sinuatrial node (pacemaker)
b Atrioventricular node
c Atrioventricular (AV) bundle (bundle of His).

The impulse for each heart beat originates at the sinuatrial node. This impulse rapidly spreads through the atria, causing contraction of these chambers, then passes through the atrioventricular node, downwards through the atrioventricular bundle to the ventricles causing ventricular contraction. The contraction phase of the heart is termed systole. The relaxation phase of the heart is termed diastole. Thus, ventricular contraction = ventricular systole. When the conducting mechanism of the heart is functioning normally – the heart is said to be in sinus rhythm.

■ The heart rate

The heart rate is controlled by the cardiac centre in the medulla and were it not for this control the sinuatrial node would cause the heart to beat at a faster rate. The vagus nerve of the parasympathetic nervous system which supplies the heart inhibits the action of the sinuatrial node maintaining it at the normal rate of approximately 70 beats per minute. The effect of the sympathetic nervous system is to increase the number of times the heart beats per minute.

■ The cardiac cycle

This is the term given to describe the events that take place in the heart during one heart beat. The event takes approximately 0.8 of a second. During this time the heart contracts and its chambers are emptied of blood, and relaxes while the chambers are filling with blood.

During diastole the atria are filling with blood, the AV valves are open, therefore some blood is passing into the ventricles. The atria contract (atrial systole (0.1 second)) filling the ventricles. The pressure inside the ventricles causes the atrioventricular valves to close, (this is the first heart sound, LUBB), and ventricular systole then occurs (0.3 second). This pushes blood out through the semilunar valves into the aorta and pulmonary artery (as the pressure inside the ventricles decreases, the AV valves open). Ventricular diastole (0.4 second) then begins and as the pressure of blood decreases in the pulmonary artery and aorta the semilunar valves shut (this is the second heart sound, DUP). Meanwhile the atria, already in diastole, are filling up with blood ready to repeat the cycle.

■ BLOOD VESSELS

The heart pumps the blood so that it may be transported around the body in tubular structures – the blood vessels.

The basic structure of arteries and veins is similar in that they consist of:
a outer connective tissue coat (tunica adventitia)
b middle smooth muscle coat (tunica media)
c inner endothelial lining (tunica intima).

■ Arteries

Arteries carry blood away from the heart. The large arteries in the body, i.e. the arteries leaving the ventricles, have a large proportion of elastic tissue in their middle coat and have great powers of recoil. The organs of the body are supplied with arteries which have been distributed by these larger arteries, they contain a large proportion of smooth muscle. These medium arteries decrease in size becoming the smallest arteries in the body – the arterioles. The area through which the blood passes is called the lumen which is small in the arteriole due to the thick layer of smooth muscle. These arteries offer resistance to the blood and help to regulate blood pressure. The flow of blood through the arteries is effected by the pumping action of the heart. The arterial blood flows from the arterioles to a network of small blood vessels called capillaries.
Note:
Arteries carry oxygenated blood, with the one exception of the pulmonary artery.

■ Capillaries

These are the smallest blood vessels in the body and are only one cell thick, i.e. an endothelial layer, and they are closely arranged around the body cells. Due to the structure of the vessel wall oxygen and nutrients can readily diffuse through to the tissue fluid and cells, and waste products can pass back through the vessel wall to be conveyed to the venous system.

■ Veins

The smallest veins in the body which receive blood from the capillary network are the venules. Blood from the venules passes into larger veins which receive tributaries and empty into the large veins which transport the blood back to the right side of the heart. The lumen of the veins are larger than those of arteries, and their walls are thinner, largely due to the

presence of fibrous tissue in the tunica media and a small amount of smooth muscle fibres. The flow of blood through the veins is smooth and the presence of valves ensures its movement in one direction. The size of the blood vessels is controlled by the vasomotor centre in the medulla.
Note:
Veins carry blood depleted in oxygen with the one exception of the pulmonary veins.

□ *Direction of the flow of blood through the circulatory system*

left side
of heart → aorta → arteries → arterioles

→ capillaries → venules → veins → superior
and vena cavae
inferior

→ right side
of heart → pulmonary artery → pulmonary
veins → left side
of heart

■ **Pulse**

The arterial pulse may be located anywhere in the body where an artery lies between the skin and a bone. The site most frequently located in practice is the radial pulse. The pulse is the wave of distension felt in an artery wall due to the contraction of the left ventricle forcing blood into the already full aorta.

■ **BLOOD PRESSURE**

Blood is ejected by the left ventricle under pressure. Blood pressure, unless qualified, refers to arterial pressure and this is the pressure exerted against the vessel wall by the blood that is pumped out by the left ventricle. The pressures recorded are those during the contraction (systolic pressure) and the relaxation of the ventricles (diastolic pressure). A sphygmomanometer is used to measure the blood pressure. This pressure is transmitted throughout the vessels in the body, but drops as the blood moves further away from the heart.

■ **Factors to consider in relation to blood pressure**

Cardiac output depends upon (a) venous return, (b) heart rate and (c) force of ventricular contraction.

Peripheral resistance depends upon (a) size of blood vessels, (b) baroreceptor activity and (c) viscosity of the blood.

Peripheral resistance is most effectively achieved by the arterioles. An increase in cardiac output or peripheral resistance brings about an increase in blood pressure.

Blood pressure is also affected by the factors which affect the activity of the vasomotor centre, such as the higher centres or any change in the levels of CO_2 and O_2 in the blood.

Adrenaline and renin increase the blood pressure by causing vasoconstriction of the arterioles.

Blood pressure varies with age and tends to increase as one gets older. An average systolic blood pressure is considered to be 120mmHg, and an average diastolic blood pressure is 80mmHg. In this case the blood pressure would be recorded as 120/80mmHg (millimetres of mercury).

■ Procedure for taking a blood pressure

The usual site for recording a blood pressure is the arm. The patient is placed in a comfortable position and an inflatable cuff is placed on the upper arm ensuring access to the cubital fossa at the elbow. The cuff is attached to the sphygmomanometer and the nurse locates the brachial pulse. She then locates the radial pulse with one hand and maintains this location while inflating the cuff with the other hand. The cuff is inflated to a point above that at which the radial pulse can no longer be felt. The stethoscope is now placed over the brachial artery and the valve is used to slowly deflate the cuff. As the column of mercury falls a sound is heard and the point at which this is heard is noted (the systolic pressure) and as the mercury continues to fall the sound becomes louder until suddenly the quality of the sound changes and becomes muffled, this point is noted as the diastolic pressure and the sounds then disappear.

■ COMMON CONDITIONS AFFECTING THE HEART AND BLOOD VESSELS INCLUDE:

■ Coronary artery disease

a Angina pectoris.
b Myocardial infarction.

The coronary arteries may become narrowed by atheroma. This narrowing may at times cause ischaemia of the myocardium giving rise to angina pectoris. The plaques of atheroma offer resistance to the blood as it passes through the coronary arteries and the likelihood of a clot's developing is increased giving rise to coronary thrombosis. A thrombus in the coronary artery may lead to occlusion and deprive an area of the myocardium of its blood supply, causing death of the myocardium. This is called a myocardial infarction.

■ **Heart failure**

Heart failure is the term used to describe the condition whereby the ventricles of the heart are not pumping sufficient blood around the body for its needs. It may involve the left ventricle only or both ventricles.
a Left ventricular failure.
b Congestive cardiac failure.

■ **Hypertension**

Describes a state where the patient's blood pressure is considered to be above normal limits. The commonest form of hypertension is essential hypertension. Malignant hypertension is relatively uncommon and causes a high mortality rate.

In approximately 10% of cases hypertension is secondary to some other disease process, e.g. renal failure.

■ **Endocarditis**

This is inflammation of the endocardium caused by organisms and/or vegetation growing on the heart valves. The Tables on pages 18–21 illustrate the important features of the above conditions.

■ DEEP VEIN THROMBOSIS

This is a condition of which nurses should always be aware as it is liable to occur as a complication of bed rest or following surgery.

■ **Factors involved**

a Stagnation of venous blood.
b A rise in blood platelet level.
c Dehydration.
d Anaemia.
e A deep vein thrombosis may be accompanied by a rise in temperature.
f Pain and tenderness of the calf.
g Swelling of the leg.
h Homan's sign may be present.
Treatment involves resting, initially avoiding active movements. Gentle physiotherapy may be given.

The patient will commence anticoagulant therapy and when over the acute stage may be allowed up with a crêpe bandage applied to the limb. Deep venous thrombosis may be prevented by encouraging a patient on bed rest to maintain movement of the legs and adequate hydration.

The complication of a deep vein thrombosis is that a part of the clot may break off and travel to the lungs – pulmonary embolism.

■ INVESTIGATIONS

■ Radiological

A chest radiograph will demonstrate any enlargement of the heart and the presence of pericardial effusion. Collection of fluid in the chest may be observed as well as calcification of the valves.

A radio-opaque substance may be introduced into the heart to enable the procedure called angiocardiography to be carried out.

■ Serum transaminase levels

SGOT: serum glutamic oxaloacetic transaminase.
SGPT: serum glutamic pyruvic transaminase.
These enzymes are released by damaged heart muscle and are elevated for the first few days following infarction.

■ Electrocardiogram (ECG) (Fig. 2)

A recording of the electrical activity in the heart muscle. Special leads are attached to the patient's limbs and chest (skin may require shaving). Some

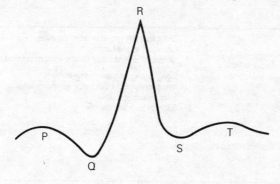

Fig. 2 The PQRST complex
P represents atrial activity
QRS represents ventricular activity
T represents the end of ventricular activity

[*cont. p. 22*]

Table A Common heart conditions:

	Angina pectoris
History	Onset usually gradual, but may be sudden
Causative factors if known	Possible factors giving rise to coronary artery disease: *i* overeating and underexercise *ii* stress and anxiety *iii* cigarette smoking *iv* hypertension *v* high intake of animal fat *vi* heredity
Clinical features	*Pain*: brought on by exertion. *Description*: gripping or constricting pain in the upper chest radiating down left arm. May radiate up to the neck or down the right arm. Sometimes pain referred to abdomen. Relieved by rest
Specific investigations	Chest radiograph Electrocardiogram
Treatment	Drug therapy aimed at relieving pain Coronary vasodilators Glyceryl trinitrate may also be used to prevent onset Long-acting coronary vasodilators Sympathetic beta blocker, e.g. propranolol Diet reducing if obese Surgery may be possible
Advice given to patients	Moderate exercise Avoid overweight/heaviness Abstain from smoking Remain in same occupation unless very stressful

Myocardial infarction	Hypertension
Onset is sudden. May be a history of angina	May be present for many years without producing symptoms
Factors as for coronary artery disease Coronary thrombosis	Unknown Heredity factors Obesity Stress Smoking
Pain: severe, may come on at rest or exertion _Description_: may be as for angina; not relieved by rest The following may also be present: A fall in blood pressure Rise in pulse rate Dyspnoea Cyanosis Temperature may be elevated	Symptoms: Left ventricular failure Cerebrovascular accident Headaches: worse in the mornings may be associated with giddiness Epistaxis Anginal pain, due to sclerotic changes in the vessels Changes may be noted in the retinal arteries Urine may contain protein
Chest radiograph Electrocardiogram SGOT: serum transaminase SGPT: levels for first 3–4 days Erythrocyte sedimentation rate (ESR)	Chest radiograph Electrocardiogram If cause of hypertension is suspected to be renal or endocrine these systems are investigated further; e.g. vanillylmandelic acid. 24-hour urine 17-ketosteroids 17-ketogenic steroids 11-hydroxycorticoids
Drug therapy: Analgesia, e.g. diamorphine Antiemetic, e.g. cyclizine Sedation, e.g. diazepam Anticoagulant therapy may be commenced (Prothrombin inhibitors) Drugs may be necessary to raise the blood pressure if hypotensive ECG monitoring of the patient for possible arrhythmias Diet: light, reducing if obese Rest: complete with gradual mobilization	If cause found it should be treated, otherwise control of hypertension is achieved by drug therapy Beta blockers Sympathetic blocking group Diuretics Ganglion blocking agents Hypertensive crisis rapid lowering of blood pressure may be necessary, e.g. ganglion blocking agent Sedation may be employed Careful recording of blood pressure: may be supine and standing. Weight reduction
As for angina Should not return to work for at least three months following the infarction	Abstain from smoking Avoid stress and anxiety Avoid becoming overweight

Table B Common heart conditions:

	Left ventricular failure (LVF)
History	Gradual or sudden
Causative factors if known	Coronary artery disease Hypertension Aortic valvular disease Mitral incompetence
Clinical features	Dyspnoea, orthopnoea Disturbed sleep, cardiac asthma may be accompanied by cough producing frothy sputum which may be blood-stained Signs of the causes of LVF may be present Hypertension Aortic valvular disease causing murmurs
Specific investigations	Chest radiograph
Treatment	Drug therapy: Sedative, e.g. morphine: reduces anxiety and hyperventilation. Diuretic, e.g. frusemide given intravenously to reduce the blood volume. Bronchial dilator, e.g. aminophylline may be given intravenously. Oxygen administration may be prescribed. Occasionally a unit of blood may be removed in an attempt to lower the venous pressure Once the acute stage is overcome the patient may require light sedation and treatment with digitalis and diuretics. Rest: position upright. Treat underlying cause if possible. Rest is followed by gradual mobilization
Advice given to patients	Will depend on patient's age and circumstances and the severity of the condition

Congestive cardiac failure	Sub-acute bacterial endocarditis (SBE)
Gradual in onset	Usually gradual onset Possibly rheumatic fever as a child causing damage to heart valves Recent dental treatment or surgery of the bowel or urinary tract
Following left ventricular failure Pulmonary embolism Congenital heart disease Disease of the mitral valve Pulmonary heart disease Thyrotoxicosis	*Streptococcus viridans*, possibly *Streptococcus faecalis* Staphylococcus
Dyspnoea and orthopnoea if pulmonary congestion is present Main signs are those caused by impairment of the venous system which empties into the rt. side of the heart Congestion in the venous system causes distension of the neck veins Liver may be enlarged with general disturbances of the gastro-intestinal tract Oedema: generalized with possibly ascites and pleural effusion Cyanosis Low urinary output containing protein	Pyrexia Later patient becomes tired and breathless and develops anaemia Vegetation may break off valve giving rise to emboli which travel to the skin causing small haemorrhages, and splinter haemorrhages under the nails Purpuric spots Kidney: red cells in the urine If large vessels are obstructed infarction can occur in any part of the body
Chest radiograph	Chest radiograph Electrocardiogram Blood culture Microscopic analysis of urine Erythrocyte sedimentation rate (ESR)
Drug therapy: Digoxin increases the cardiac and reduces the venous pressure. Diuretics are also employed to lower the venous pressure (potassium supplements) Sedation may be required if patient is anxious and restless Oxygen may be required and if the patient has a lung disease the concentration of oxygen is prescribed Rest: Bed and chair. Position upright with legs lowered to allow oedema fluid to drain away from the lungs. Prevent any strain on the heart Use of commode Prevention of constipation Measure urinary output/rest Diet: light, and reduction of salt intake Weigh patient daily Collection of oedema in the abdomen or chest may be mechanically removed	Drug therapy: appropriate antibiotic is prescribed for the causative organism and is continued for a number of weeks. May initially be given by means of intravenous infusion Rest in bed is maintained until patient's general condition is improved
As for left ventricular failure	As for failure

electrodes require the application of electrode jelly to increase the effectiveness of transmission. It is possible to obtain intermittent graph readings, or a cardiac monitor may be used for continuous observation of the heart's activity. The reading obtained by the ECG is represented by the PQRST complex.

Routine investigations would be carried out as well as the specific ones mentioned.

■ SUMMARY OF THE NURSING CARE FOR PATIENTS WITH DISEASES AFFECTING THE HEART

The fact that a patient has a cardiac condition is the cause of much anxiety to both the patient and his family, and all will require information and explanation of treatment and investigations as well as reassurance. Rest of varying degrees is necessary during the course of treatment for most cardiac conditions. This is achieved by a calm, quiet environment and the avoidance of any activity and excitement that will tire the patient. It may be necessary for sedation to be prescribed to help the patient to sleep.

■ Position

Position of the patient is related to the specific condition; generally though, if the patient is dyspnoeic (as in heart failure) he is better sitting up well supported with pillows.

■ Eating and drinking

The dietician may be involved to discuss problems with the patient. For coronary artery disease, diet may have to be low in animal fat and cholesterol. Salt is restricted for heart failure when accompanied by oedema. In most cases diet should be light and easily digestible. In some instances the patient may require help with feeding. Intravenous infusion may be necessary either to maintain the hydration of the patient or for the administration of drugs. For instance, the antibiotics prescribed in subacute bacterial endocarditis, and drugs used for the correction of arrhythmias which may arise following a myocardial infarction. All intravenous fluids would be prescribed by the doctor. The nurse, however, should be aware of circulatory overloading and observe the patient closely. The patient's skin should be warm and dry and the normal colour for the patient, and vital observations should be checked regularly by the nurse.

All fluids should be recorded on a fluid balance chart. All intravenous fluid should be checked before being given and the patient must be identified. Also check the fluid container for the expiry date. Urinary output should be recorded. The nurse should ensure that the prescribed infusion is flowing at the correct rate, that the tubing remains patent and that the cannula site is checked regularly. Batch number should be recorded on fluid balance chart. The splint should be comfortable and the hand and/or arm observed for swelling, pain or inflammation. Any abnormalities should be reported.

All fluids administered should be recorded and an accurate fluid balance chart should be maintained so that the effects of diuretics in heart failure, for example, can be monitored. The patient may also be weighed daily so that an assessment of the response of oedema to therapy can be made.

■ Elimination

Constipation should be avoided in patients with heart conditions so as to prevent strain on the heart and to avoid abdominal distension which may further embarrass the patient's breathing. A commode is often less of a strain for patients than a bedpan. Urinary output should be recorded; a low urinary output may be indicative of cardiac failure developing as a complication to some other heart condition.

Urine may have to be tested for protein in cases of heart failure and hypertension. It is tested for blood if the patient is receiving anticoagulant therapy.

■ Drugs

These are administered as prescribed and the nurse should have some knowledge of the action and possible side-effects of the drugs so that she may effectively observe the patient's response to treatment.

■ Pain

Many heart conditions give rise to pain. As well as administering the analgesics prescribed, the nurse should be aware of the other factors which may be associated with the patient's ability to cope with pain (see *Principles of Nursing* in this series).

■ Mobilization

Patients with a heart condition require rest, possibly in bed, and the nurse will have to assess carefully the patient's requirements, so that pressure sore formation is avoided. It is important to state clearly the extent of activity that the patient is allowed in terms of washing, moving, shaving, etc., so that the heart is receiving adequate rest. The physiotherapist is involved with the mobilization programme for the patient, which will involve chest physiotherapy for patients with pulmonary oedema as a result of heart failure, and leg exercises for the prevention of deep venous thrombosis.

If possible, suitable diversional and occupational therapy may be given.

■ **Advice on discharge**

The advice that is given to patients prior to their discharge has to be considered in the light of the patient's lifestyle, occupation, the severity of the condition and his understanding of the illness.

■ **PRACTICE QUESTIONS**

1 *What is meant by the following terms?*
   a Endocardium.
   b Properties of rhythmicity and conductivity.
   c Cardiac output.
   d Sinuatrial node.
   e Ventricular diastole.
   f Cardiac centre.
   g Cardiac cycle.
   h Heart sounds.
   i Pulse.
   j Blood pressure.
   k Peripheral resistance.
   l Angina pectoris.
   m Myocardial infarction.
   n Atheroma.
   o Ischaemia.
   p Coronary thrombosis.
   q Sclerotic changes.
   r Coronary vasodilators.
   s Electrocardiogram.
   t Anticoagulant therapy.
   u Sympathetic beta blockers.
   v Oedema.
   w Orthopnoea.
   x Antibiotic.
   y Diuretic.

z Homan's sign.
aa Valvular incompetence.
bb Valvular stenosis.
cc Hypertension.
dd Embolism.

2 *Briefly explain the following:*

a The mechanism of conduction through the heart.
b The direction of blood flow through the body beginning at the atrium.
c The formation of tissue fluid.
d Why tissue fluid is not normally produced in the lungs.
e The possible causes of oedema in congestive cardiac failure.
f Why peripheral resistance is most effectively achieved by the arterioles.
g The pathway for the transmission of sympathetic nerve impulses from the vasomotor centre to the arterioles.
h The underlying physiology causing the pain on effort experienced by patients with angina pectoris.
i The signs of digoxin toxicity.
j Coronary artery disease.

3 *Mark the following statements true or false:*

a An electrocardiogram is performed following a myocardial infarction to determine the extent and location of the infarction.
b A sympathetic beta-blocking agent should not be given to patients with asthma as it causes constriction of the bronchioles.
c Right-sided heart failure is always caused by left-sided failure.
d The baroreceptors are sensitive to the pressure of blood inside the arteries.
e Vasodilation of the arterioles increases the peripheral resistance.
f The cardiac centre controls the size of blood vessels.
g Valves are found in veins so that the blood will flow in one direction only.
h The antidote for warfarin is vitamin K.
i Tissue fluid is formed at the arterial end of the capillary.
j The pulmonary artery carries oxygenated blood away from the heart.
k The heart sounds are produced by the opening of the atrioventricular and semilunar valves.
l Hypertension can eventually cause hypertrophy of the left ventricle.
m Coupled heart beats may be a sign of digoxin overdose.
n The presence of a swelling in the calf is termed Homan's sign.
o Cardiac output is usually reduced in cardiac failure.
p Hypertension is not a disease which runs in families.

q Renin is an enzyme which is produced by the kidneys in response to an inadequate blood flow, and it acts on a substance in the plasma to produce angiotensin which causes an increase in blood pressure by causing vasoconstriction of the arterioles.

r Due to the amount of fibrous tissue in the tunica media of the vein the lumen is larger than that of the artery.

s The P wave on an ECG reflects atrial activity.

t Following a myocardial infarction the erythrocyte sedimentation rate usually remains unchanged.

4 *Attempt to answer the following question*
(A guide is given as to the information which should be included, in the answer section.)
Mr Brown is a 43-year-old managing director admitted to your ward following a myocardial infarction while away from home on a business trip for his company. He is married with three young children of school age. Describe the total care and management of Mr Brown while he is in hospital.

■ **Answers**

1 *a* Interior surface of the heart (squamous epithelium).

b Rhythmicity: alternately contracts and relaxes rhythmically from one fibre to the other. Conductivity: the ability to conduct impulses.

c The blood ejected by each ventricle every minute.

d Situated in the right atrium close to the entrance of the superior vena cava. Heart beat originates at the SA node which is known as the pacemaker.

e The ventricles are in a state of relaxation.

f Special cells found in the medulla which control the heart rate. The cardiac centre in turn receives impulses from different parts of the body.

g The series of events which take place during a heart beat.

h Sounds produced by the heart which may be heard through a stethoscope. They are produced by closure of the atrioventricular and semilunar valves.

i A wave of distension which may be felt in the artery in a part of the body where the artery runs over a bone near to the skin surface.

j The pressure which is exerted against the walls of the arteries by the blood being pumped out of the left ventricle.

k The resistance offered to blood as it passes through the arterioles particularly (due to the smaller lumen) and helps to regulate the blood pressure.

l A disease characterized by chest pain on exertion due to inadequate oxygen supplies reaching the myocardium.

m When a part of the myocardium dies because the blood supply to the part has been stopped.

n Changes which take place in the arterial walls, causing thickening and the development of plaques on the intima, thought to be caused by cholesterol and other lipids.

o Ischaemia is the term used when an organ or muscle is not receiving an adequate blood supply.

p The presence of a clot in the coronary arteries.

q Changes that take place which are largely degenerative and due to the process of ageing.

r Drugs that are used to dilate the coronary arteries.

s An investigation to trace the electrical impulses given off by the heart.

t Anticoagulant therapy involves the administration of drugs which will interfere with the normal blood clotting mechanism, thereby reducing the coagulability of the blood.

u They will block the response of beta receptors to adrenaline. In response to stress, for example, the heart is stimulated by increasing the heart rate, this response is inhibited by the use of sympathetic beta blockers.

v The presence of excessive tissue fluid.

w Difficulty in breathing when lying down.

x Drugs that are antibacterial in action and are prescribed for disease caused by various organisms.

y Drugs given to increase the urinary output.

z Pain in the calf produced by dorsiflexion of the foot.

aa Improper closure of heart valves.

bb Inadequate outlet through the valves.

cc A high blood pressure.

dd A particle being carried through the circulation by the blood, may be a piece of clot from a thrombosis, air or fat.

2 *a* Impulses originate at the sinuatrial node and pass in an orderly fashion through the atria causing them to contract (to the atrioventricular node) down the atrioventricular bundle and up through the ventricles bringing about ventricular contraction.

b Left atrium → left ventricle → aorta → arterial branches → capillaries → veins → right atrium → right ventricle → pulmonary artery → lungs → pulmonary veins → left atrium.

   c Tissue fluid is formed at the arterial end of the capillary because the blood pressure (32mmHg) is greater than the osmotic pressure (25mmHg) exerted by the plasma proteins. Thus, water is forced out into the tissue spaces. At the venous end of the capillary the blood pressure has dropped (12mmHg) and is less than the osmotic pressure. This has the effect of taking in tissue fluid to the capillary from the tissue spaces.

   d Because the pressure in the pulmonary blood vessels and capillaries is usually lower then the osmotic force exerted by the plasma proteins.

   e *i* An increase in venous pressure preventing the re-absorption of tissue fluid.

      ii Stagnant anoxia causing the release of renin by the kidneys resulting in the formation of angiotensin which stimulates the production of aldosterone with subsequent retention of sodium and water.

   f The lumen of the arteriole is small because of the thick layer of smooth muscle, the amount of blood passing through them can be reduced by decreasing the size of the lumen. This has the effect of blood damming in the systemic arteries raising the blood pressure.

   g The transmission is achieved by three neurones. The first neurone runs from the vasomotor centre in the medulla down to the lateral horn cells of grey matter in the spinal cord. The second neurone runs from the spinal cord to the sympathetic (autonomic) ganglion (preganglionic fibre). The third neurone runs from the ganglion to the blood vessels (the postganglionic fibre).

   h Muscular activity produces metabolites. An increased blood flow is required to remove these metabolites. If the blood flow is inadequate pain will develop.

   i Nausea, vomiting, diarrhoea, coupled beats, excessive slowing of the pulse.

   j Changes take place in the arteries; initially they become hardened due to plaques of atheroma, eventually the supply of blood to the myocardium is impaired giving rise to ischaemia, the vessels may become further occluded by the development of thrombi, depriving the myocardium of its blood supply.

3 *a* True   *f* False   *k* False   *p* False
   b True   *g* True   *l* True   *q* True
   c False   *h* True   *m* True   *r* True
   d True   *i* True   *n* False   *s* True
   e False   *j* False   *o* True   *t* False

4 The following points should be included in the answer:

a Patient's position in the ward; close observation, possibly a coronary care unit.

b Hard base to the bed, fracture board.

c Space for accommodating equipment, cardiac monitor, intravenous stands.

d Calm, quiet atmosphere.

e Position in bed, comfort, bearing in mind patient's condition, adequate pillows.

f Emergency admission, inform relatives, care of patient's property.

g Observations: temperature, pulse, respirations, and blood pressure as frequently as patient's condition requires. Cardiac monitor for arrhythmias.
Observation of skin care and texture, fluid balance, urinary output.
Observation and maintenance of intravenous infusion.

h Administration of analgesia, antiemetic, oxygen, anticoagulants as prescribed.

i Providing support and reassurance for the patient during procedures and investigations; blood investigations, radiological examination of the chest, electrocardiogram.

j Eating and drinking: fluids may be offered as desired, diet when the patient can tolerate it should be light and easily digestible.

k Elimination: urine should be routinely tested. Tested for blood if anticoagulant therapy is prescribed; check output. Bowels: prevent constipation and straining. The use of a commode may cause less distress than a bedpan.

l Mobilization: complete bed rest for 1st 24–48 hours – gentle physiotherapy. Adequate number of nurses to lift, move and change patient's position. Prevent sore formation. Active participation of the patient is gradual. Time spent up in chair gradually increased from ½ hour to 1 hour to 2 hours daily.

m Skin and general hygiene: patient participation is gradual. Bedbaths initially then assisted washing, eventually patient can manage himself. Shaving performed by nurses while patient on complete bed rest. Care of hair and nails. Oral hygiene, provide facilities for cleaning teeth, keep mouth moist.

n Accommodation may have to be provided for the wife. Involvement of extended family to help with children, involvement of medical social worker. Allow wife to discuss anxieties. Keep patient informed regarding children, e.g. photographs. Advice regarding convalescence, stress, diet, smoking.

3 Blood

The objectives of this section are to:

1 Describe the composition of blood.
2 Identify factors necessary for the clotting of blood.
3 Explain the blood grouping system and the care required by patients receiving a blood transfusion.
4 Identify common diseases affecting the blood.
5 Describe the investigations and total management of patients with the above diseases.

■ CHARACTERISTICS OF BLOOD

The body contains approximately 5 litres of blood which is transported around the body in the blood vessels. Oxygen, nutrients, waste products, carbon dioxide, hormones, enzymes, immunoglobulins (antibodies) and plasma proteins are all carried around the body by the blood. It is slightly alkaline with a pH of 7.4 which is maintained by the kidneys, lungs and the buffer systems. Blood is composed of cells and plasma. This can be illustrated by obtaining a specimen of blood, placing it in a tube containing an anticoagulant and allowing it to stand. It will be seen to separate out into layers, the cells sinking to the bottom and the plasma remaining above as a yellow-coloured fluid; 45% of the blood volume is made up of red cells and this figure constitutes the haematocrit (or the packed cell volume (PCV)). There is a slight variation in the normal range between males and females.

■ BLOOD CELLS

■ Erythrocytes (red blood cells)

In every cubic millimetre of blood there are 5 million red blood cells (SI measurement – 4.5×10^{12}/litre). Each cell is a biconcave disc 7 microns in diameter and 2 microns thick. Each cell contains the pigment haemoglobin which carries the oxygen. When combined with oxygen it is a bright red colour and is known as oxyhaemoglobin: without oxygen it is a dark blue colour and is known as reduced haemoglobin. Each 100ml of blood contains approximately 14.8g (g/dl) of haemoglobin. Fully developed circulating red blood cells have no nuclei. They are formed in the red bone marrow from the stem cell. The process of formation of red blood cells is called erythropoiesis.

□ *Erythropoiesis*

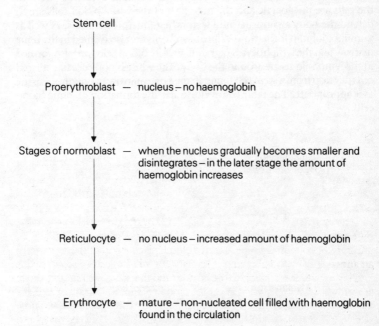

Stem cell

Proerythroblast — nucleus – no haemoglobin

Stages of normoblast — when the nucleus gradually becomes smaller and disintegrates – in the later stage the amount of haemoglobin increases

Reticulocyte — no nucleus – increased amount of haemoglobin

Erythrocyte — mature – non-nucleated cell filled with haemoglobin found in the circulation

Factors necessary for the formation of red blood cells include the presence of erythropoietin (a substance produced by the kidney which stimulates production of red blood cells). Dietary factors are also important (protein, vitamins C and B_{12}, folic acid, iron, traces of copper) and a healthy bone marrow.

The red blood cells live for about 120 days after which they are destroyed by the phagocytic cells of the reticulo-endothelial system. The iron is removed, stored and used to form new blood cells. The remainder of the haem portion is converted to bile pigments, bilirubin and biliverdin which are excreted in faeces via the liver and biliary tract. The protein (globin) is retained as amino acids for further use by the body.

■ **Leucocytes** (white blood cells)

There are between 5000 and 10 000 white blood cells per cubic millimetre (SI measurement $4.0-10.0 \times 10^9$/litre) of blood. There are many different types of white blood cells which are classified according to whether or not there are granules present in the cytoplasm of the cell. White blood cells are slightly larger in size than red cells and contain a nucleus. Many of the cells are phagocytic and the functions of the white blood cells are to defend the body against harmful factors, e.g. micro-organisms, as well as immunoglobulin formation. White blood cells are also formed in the bone marrow and the lymphocytes (agranular white blood cells) are also formed in the lymphoid tissue around the body. The white blood cells like the red cells develop from a stem cell found in the bone marrow or lymphoid tissue as is appropriate. The table below illustrates the formation of white blood cells.

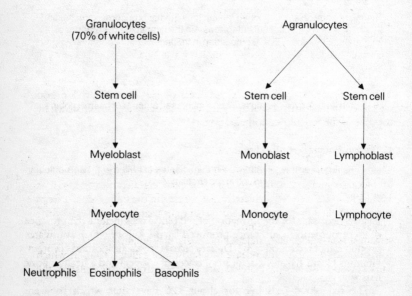

□ *Granulocytes*
The nuclei of the granulocytes have several lobes.

Neutrophils defend the body against infection and have the ability to move out through the capillary wall into the tissues when necessary; this is called diapedesis. Neutrophils are numerous and constitute the largest proportion of the granulocytes. They are also phagocytic and when they have been used up, in the process of bacterial destruction for example, they die. Pus contains a large number of dead neutrophils.

Eosinophils increase in number in response to allergic states such as asthma and hay fever and assume antihistamine properties. They also increase in number in response to worm infestation. The lobules of the nuclei are not as distinctive as those of the neutrophils. They live for between 12 and 20 hours.

Basophils are very small in number and produce heparin and histamine. The lobules of the nuclei are even less distinctive than those of the other granulocytes.

Monocytes are the largest of the white blood cells and are phagocytic. They are considerably fewer in number than the lymphocytes and contain a kidney-shaped nucleus.

Lymphocytes increase in number in response to chronic infections, i.e. infections which persist for a reasonable length of time. Lymphocytes also produce immunoglobulins. Lymphocytes are of different sizes and contain large nuclei. Their life span varies, depending on type, from a few hours to 200 days.

The factors necessary for the production of red blood cells are also necessary for the formation of the white cells. The cells are broken down by the cells of the reticulo-endothelial system.

■ Thrombocytes or blood platelets

These are the smallest of all the blood cells and each cubic millimetre of blood contains 250 000 to 500 000 platelets (SI measurement is $150-400 \times 10^9$/litre). The platelets are formed in the bone marrow from large cells called megakaryocytes. It is thought that the cytoplasm of the megakaryocytes (which are nucleated) breaks off and enters the blood-stream as non-nucleated platelets. These cells play an important role in the formation of a clot by the release of a substance called serotonin which causes vasoconstriction. Platelets are also destroyed by cells of the reticulo-endothelial system.

■ Plasma

91% of plasma is made up of water; the remaining 9% consists of solids such as nutrients; waste products, including carbon dioxide; inorganic salts, hormones, enzymes and immunoglobulins.

Plasma proteins are also contained in plasma. These are formed in the liver and are:

Albumin
Globulin
Fibrinogen
Prothrombin.

☐ *Functions of plasma proteins*
1 Providing viscosity to the blood.
2 Buffering action, i.e. they help to maintain a blood pH of 7.4.
3 Immunoglobulins are mainly carried by the globulin.
4 Osmotic pressure. Plasma proteins are unable to pass through the capillary wall and are therefore important in the formation and absorption of tissue fluid because of the osmotic pressure they exert.
5 Transport. Many substances circulating in the blood are carried by the plasma proteins, e.g. lipids which are insoluble in water.
6 Blood clotting. Fibrinogen and prothrombin are necessary for clot formation.

☐ *Blood clotting* (See chart p. 35)
Blood circulating in normal healthy blood vessels does not usually clot, unless there is damage to the vessel walls which may trap platelets, which may in turn form a clot. While the clot is contained in the vessel it is known as a thrombus. If the thrombus or a part of it becomes detached and moves freely in the circulation it is termed an embolus. If blood is removed or leaves the blood vessels it will form a clot within a few minutes.

Other factors present in plasma are involved in the formation of thromboplastin. They include Factor VIII (antihaemophilic globulin) and Factor IX (Christmas factor). Absence of these factors will produce haemophilia or Christmas disease.

■ BLOOD GROUPS

A person's blood group is determined by the ABO system. The blood group to which a person belongs is determined by the presence or absence of **agglutinogens** (antigens) carried on the surface of the red blood cell. The letters A and B are used to describe the agglutinogens.

The presence of agglutinogen A – blood group A
The presence of agglutinogen B – blood group B
The presence of both agglutinogens A and B – blood group AB
The absence of both agglutinogens – blood group O

Factors necessary for the formation of a clot

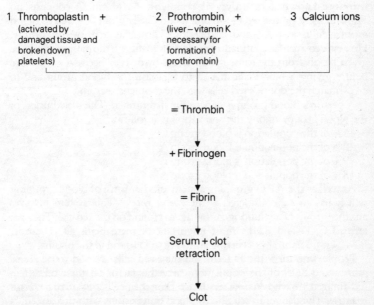

1 Thromboplastin + (activated by damaged tissue and broken down platelets)

2 Prothrombin + (liver – vitamin K necessary for formation of prothrombin)

3 Calcium ions

= Thrombin

+ Fibrinogen

= Fibrin

Serum + clot retraction

Clot

Naturally occurring antibodies called **agglutinins** are present in the plasma, so that a person who is blood group A (due to the presence of agglutinogen A on the red cell) would have the anti-B agglutinin in the plasma. The presence of agglutinins in relation to the blood group would be as follows:

Red cell (agglutinogens)	Blood group	Plasma (agglutinins)
A	A	anti-B
B	B	anti-A
AB	AB	**no** agglutinins
no agglutinogens	O	anti-A and anti-B

It can therefore be seen that blood group A cannot be given to a patient who is blood group B, because the agglutinin (anti-A) in the plasma of the person receiving the blood would cause agglutination (clumping) of the donor's red blood cells which contain agglutinogen A. Theoretically it can be seen that blood group AB, because it contains no agglutinins (anti-A –

anti-B) in the plasma, can receive blood from groups A, B and O and is therefore known as a **universal recipient**. As group O contains no agglutinogens on the red blood cell, theoretically it can be given to blood groups A, B and AB and is therefore known as a **universal donor**. However to avoid agglutination during a transfusion the patient would be given blood from the same group as his own. It is necessary therefore before giving a blood transfusion to establish the blood group and to cross-match the donor's red cells with the recipient's serum.

A person's blood group is genetically determined. The distribution of the blood groups among the population is as follows:

46% of the population is blood group O

42% of the population is blood group A

9% of the population is blood group B

3% of the population is blood group AB

As well as the ABO grouping system another form of blood grouping which has to be considered is the *rhesus system*. This system involves another group of agglutinogens (antigens) found on the red cell. They are termed C, D and E, the most important of them being D. There is, however, no naturally occurring antibody to D found in the plasma.

People who carry the D factor on their red cells are said to be *rhesus positive* and 85% of the population carry this factor on their cells. The remaining 15% who do not carry factor D on their cells are said to be *rhesus negative*. The danger in relation to blood transfusions with this system is that should a person who is rhesus negative receive rhesus positive blood, he will produce antibodies (anti-D) which will cause agglutination of the rhesus positive cells. A rhesus positive person cannot produce anti-D antibodies and they can therefore receive rhesus negative blood. The formation of anti-D may also occur in the rhesus negative pregnant woman carrying a rhesus positive baby who has inherited the D factor from the father. The anti-D produced by the mother will cause agglutination of the baby's red cells, if any of the baby's blood enters the mother's circulation. It is the presence of the D factor in the baby's blood that stimulates the production of anti-D in the mother's blood. Exchange transfusion with rhesus negative blood may be necessary once the baby has been born. As the rhesus factor is genetically inherited the baby will later make his own rhesus positive cells, by which time the anti-D in his circulation will have disappeared.

■ BLOOD TRANSFUSIONS

It is important for the nurse to be familiar with the policy governing the collection and setting up of blood.

It is usual for two people to check the following before the blood transfusion is commenced, and at least one of them should be a trained nurse or doctor:

1 The patient's name, age, and address, verbally if possible; the identity bracelet on the patient is also checked.
2 The ABO group and rhesus factor.
3 The serial number and expiry date of the blood being used.

All details should correspond with the patient's notes. Blood should not be collected from the blood bank until needed. The correct procedure is followed for the collection of blood from the bank and the blood is signed for.

■ Possible complications of blood transfusions

1 Simple reaction to a foreign protein (donor blood). There may be a transient rise in temperature, headache, and an increase in pulse rate. The transfusion is slowed and the doctor is informed.
2 An allergic reaction is caused by hypersensitivity to a foreign protein. There may be headache and nausea, accompanied by an urticarial rash. The transfusion is slowed and the doctor informed; he may prescribe antihistamine drugs.
3 Incompatibility occurs as a result of mis-match of the ABO or rhesus group in the blood transfusion. The patient may complain of severe pain in the loin. There may be nausea and vomiting, shivering and restlessness, and the patient's skin may be cold and clammy. There may also be a rise in the patient's temperature, increased pulse and respiration rates and, as the patient becomes shocked, the blood pressure will fall. Observation of temperature, pulse, respirations, and blood pressure should be carried out at f. equent regular intervals and the patient should be closely observed throughout the transfusion. There may also be a reduction in the urinary output and urine should be tested for protein. The doctor should be informed immediately and the transfusion stopped. The treatment given will depend on the patient's condition and may involve the administration of intravenous hydrocortisone. Air embolism may be a complication but the incidence is greatly reduced by the use of plastic floats and collapsible bags.

Thrombophlebitis may cause pain and inflammation of the affected vein; if it occurs the cannula is removed and an alternative site is selected.

If a blood transfusion is preceded or followed by intravenous fluids, a different giving set should be used.

It is important that the blood is given at the rate prescribed by the doctor.

Blood may have to be heated during the course of a transfusion if a pump is being used.

A record should be kept of all blood transfused and if more than one unit of blood is given, the collecting and checking procedure must be followed for each subsequent unit. The procedure for the disposal of blood bags must be correctly followed. If a reaction to the blood occurs it is usual for the bag to be returned to the laboratory for investigation. It is usual, however, for all bags to be retained on the ward for 24 hours following a transfusion. The patient should be kept comfortable during the course of the transfusion and all care should be taken by the nurses when handling blood bags.

The common conditions which affect the blood include the anaemias and leukaemias.

■ ANAEMIA

Anaemia is said to be present when there is a reduction in the number of red blood cells and the oxygen-carrying substance haemoglobin. Many of the signs and symptoms of anaemia result from the body's inability to carry sufficient oxygen around the body, and the degree of manifestation will depend on the severity of the anaemia. Signs include:

a dizziness, faintness, headaches
b pallor of the mucous membranes
c tiredness
d anorexia and dyspepsia
e tingling and 'pins and needles' in the extremities
e tachycardia and palpitations
f breathlessness on exertion
g possibly oedema and angina in the older person.

■ Causes of anaemia

Anaemia may be due to:

1 The inability to produce normal red blood cells because the factors necessary for their formation are inadequate.
2 Having been formed the blood cells are lost through haemorrhage.
3 The destruction of the red blood cells exceeds the body's ability to form them.

□ *Anaemia due to deficiency of erythropoietic factors*
a Iron deficiency anaemia
This is the most common of all the anaemias. Iron is found in foods such as meat, eggs, cheese and cabbage; it is not present in milk. Iron is necessary for the formation of haemoglobin and deficiency may occur due to inadequate dietary intake, blood loss or gastric hypochlorhydria (hydrochloric acid is necessary for the absorption of iron). Deficiency may also be due to an increased demand for iron by the body, as occurs in women during the childbearing years, due to blood loss during menstruation and due to the nutritional demands of pregnancy and lactation.

As well as the signs and symptoms already mentioned the patient may also experience:
Soreness of the mouth and tongue.
Tongue may be smooth and red due to atrophy of the papillae.
Dysphagia.
The group of symptoms described above, combined with iron deficiency anaemia, are together known as the Plummer-Vinson syndrome. Koilonychia may also be present.

Investigations include a blood examination including a full blood count, red cell count and measurement of the haemoglobin content of erythrocytes (the cells are microcytic and hypochromic). More specific tests may include measuring the:
  i Haematocrit value.
  ii Mean corpuscular haemoglobin (MCH): amount of haemoglobin in each cell.
  iii Mean corpuscular haemoglobin concentration (MCHC): haemoglobin concentration in the cells.
  iv Mean corpuscular volume (MCV): the volume of the cells.

Other investigations may be necessary to determine the possible cause of anaemia; for example it may be caused by chronic bleeding which may not be visible to the naked eye, or it may be due to a peptic ulcer or a malignant disease.

The treatment for iron deficiency anaemia includes a well balanced diet containing iron-rich food, as well as the administration of medicinal iron. It may be given orally, for example in the form of ferrous sulphate taken after meals. Iron preparations are also available in syrup form. Vitamin C may also be prescribed. If for some reason oral preparations cannot be taken the physician may prescribe an intramuscular preparation, e.g. Imferon. It is sometimes considered necessary for the patient to receive a blood transfusion.

□ *Nursing care*

The specific nursing care will depend on many factors, such as the patient's age and condition. Generally, however, if the patient's haemoglobin level is very low the physician may recommend complete bed rest and the nurse would have to consider all the factors in relation to mobility, aids used for the prevention of sores, the maintenance of general hygiene, and the condition of skin, hair and nails. She should provide support and reassurance for the patient during the course of investigations.

She should observe the degree of pallor of the mucous membranes and carry out specific observations required by the doctor. She should ensure that the patient receives the correct diet, that the diet is taken and that medication is taken and that medication is administered as prescribed. Oral liquid preparations containing iron are best given through a straw to avoid staining the patient's teeth. Careful attention should be paid to the patient's mouth and the doctor may prescribe an oral antiseptic mouthwash to treat soreness.

All aspects of care should be explained to the patient, including the fact that the stools may be black due to the administration of the iron preparation. Iron may also cause constipation and it may be necessary to give the patient a mild aperient.

Whether the patient is on complete bed rest or not, the achievement of adequate rest, sleep and relaxation is important.

b Anaemia due to vitamin B_{12} and folic acid deficiency

Vitamin B_{12} (cyanocobalamin), known as the extrinsic factor, is stored in the liver and is transported to the bone marrow as necessary for the normal maturation of red blood cells. Vitamin B_{12} is found in foods containing proteins. The gastric glands in the stomach produce a substance which is necessary for the absorption of vitamin B_{12} in the terminal ileum. This substance is termed the intrinsic factor. The absence of the intrinsic factor in the gastric juice is associated with the absence of hydrochloric acid. Vitamin B_{12} is also necessary for the formation of another B vitamin called folic acid.

Vitamin B_{12} deficiency may develop due to an inadequate dietary intake (rare in Britain); failure of the stomach to produce sufficient intrinsic factor (Addisonian pernicious anaemia); following gastrectomy; disease of the intestinal tract or disease of the liver. Vitamin B_{12} is also needed by the cells of the nervous system and a deficiency may lead to the condition of subacute combined degeneration of the spinal cord. This condition, not hypochlorhydria, is manifested in B_{12} deficiencies due to inadequate dietary intake, intestinal or liver disease. Treatment of B_{12} deficiency other than that caused by the lack of intrinsic factor includes parenteral administration of vitamin B_{12}; folic acid may also be prescribed and the cause, if known, is treated. The commonest vitamin B_{12} deficiency is pernicious anaemia. It is more common in women than men and there is a familial tendency. The red blood cells are larger than normal (macrocytic) and irregular in shape. It is unusual before the age of 30 years.

As well as the general signs and symptoms of anaemia (see page 38) the patient may have:

   i Loss of weight (may not be significant).

   ii Loss of appetite.

   iii Sore tongue (red and raw appearance, ulcers may be present).

   iv Skin may show a faint lemon-yellow tint (due to rapid breakdown of abnormal red cells).

   v Abdominal pain and diarrhoea.

   vi Neurological symptoms may be present.

In addition to the blood investigations (see page 39) the following may be carried out:

   i Estimation of serum level of vitamin B_{12}.

   ii Gastric analysis test to determine the presence or otherwise of hydrochloric acid in the stomach. This involves fasting the patient, usually overnight, passing a nasogastric tube, the administration of a gastric secretory stimulant, e.g. pentagastrin, and the aspiration of the stomach contents at stated intervals. All specimen containers should be correctly labelled.

   iii Bone marrow puncture so that a specimen of the bone marrow may be obtained for laboratory examination.

   iv Schilling test. This involves the oral administration of B_{12} labelled with radio-active cobalt, followed by an intramuscular administration of ordinary vitamin B_{12}. A 24-hour collection of urine is obtained and an estimation of the radio-active vitamin B_{12} contained in the urine is made.

When a diagnosis of pernicious anaemia is made the patient is given intramuscular injections of vitamin B_{12} preparation, e.g. hydroxocobalamin, and it is explained to the patient that he will require regular maintenance doses for the rest of his life. Blood will be obtained at regular intervals so that the patient's response to treatment can be monitored. Iron therapy may also be necessary at the commencement of treatment due to the rapid regeneration of red blood cells in response to the vitamin B_{12} replacement. Diet should be light, well balanced, rich in protein, iron and vitamins.

It may be considered necessary for the patient to receive a blood transfusion. As in all types of long-standing anaemia blood is given slowly, as a sudden increase in blood volume may cause heart failure.

Following discharge from hospital the patient will continue to receive vitamin B_{12} injections every four to eight weeks. Regular blood counts are performed at six-monthly intervals and the patient attends the outpatient department so that his condition is continuously monitored.

The nursing care for the patient admitted to hospital with pernicious anaemia follows the same lines as that for iron deficiency anaemia, taking into account the individual needs of each patient.

Other anaemias caused by deficiency of erythropoietic factors are those due to vitamin C (ascorbic acid) deficiency. Such deficiencies are associated with scurvy which is caused by insufficient protein, minerals and ascorbic acid in the diet. Treatment is a well-balanced diet containing fruit and vegetables; vitamin C supplements may be ordered. Iron is also given when anaemia is associated with iron deficiency. Deficiency of thyroxine may also cause anaemia and is associated with myxoedema. The treatment involves the administration of thyroxine and any accompanying iron deficiency is appropriately treated.

c Aplastic anaemia (pancytopenia)

This anaemia develops when there is decreased activity in the bone marrow, resulting in insufficient production of leucocytes and thrombocytes as well as the red blood cells. The cause of aplastic anaemia may be unknown (idiopathic) or depression of the bone marrow activity may be caused by certain drugs, chemicals, over-exposure to *x*-rays or radio-active materials.

Treatment of the patient is in relation to the severity of the condition and, if possible, the cause is removed. Transfusions are given as and when required, antibiotics are administered to combat infections and the patient is closely observed for bleeding from different parts of the body. Prednisolone may be prescribed and reverse barrier nursing may be employed.

□ *Anaemia due to loss of blood through haemorrhage*

Loss of blood may be acute or chronic. An acute haemorrhage usually means the loss of a considerable volume of blood over a short period of time. Chronic haemorrhage is loss of small amounts of blood, usually over a period of time, e.g. as occurs with haemorrhoids, menorrhagia, peptic ulcer. In anaemia due to chronic haemorrhage it is necessary to find the cause and administer iron to treat the anaemia. The sudden loss of a large volume of blood, as in acute haemorrhage, may require a blood transfusion to reverse the state of shock and, during the recovery period, iron therapy may be necessary. As haemodilution takes some hours to develop following the loss of blood from the circulatory system, the decrease in haemoglobin level will not be reflected immediately following haemorrhage.

□ *Anaemia due to the excessive destruction of red blood cells* (haemolytic anaemia)

As stated earlier, red blood cells are destroyed by the cells of the reticuloendothelial system and when the rate of destruction exceeds the rate of formation by the bone marrow a haemolytic anaemia develops. It may be caused by congenital abnormalities of the erythrocytes, many of which are spherical in shape and fragile, or due to the presence of abnormal haemoglobins.

Other causes of haemolytic anaemia include micro-organisms, e.g. haemolytic streptococci; agents such as arsenic, lead and sulphonamides; the formation of erythrocyte antibodies as in haemolytic disease of the newborn; or a person may develop antibodies which destroy his own red blood cells as in autoimmune haemolytic anaemia. Transfusion with incompatible blood also causes haemolysis of the donor's red cells.

In addition to the signs and symptoms of anaemia, the excessive breakdown of red blood cells causes an increase in the level of serum bilirubin, giving rise to jaundice. Urobilinogen is also present in the urine. In an attempt to meet the demand for red cells the body produces immature cells, so that there is an increase in the number of circulating reticulocytes (see p. 31). The treatment for the haemolytic anaemias is dependent on the severity of the symptoms manifested by the patient, and ranges from blood transfusions and administration of steroids to splenectomy, depending on the cause of haemolysis.

■ SUMMARY OF NURSING CARE REQUIRED BY PATIENTS WHO ARE ANAEMIC

The nursing care required by patients will be based on individual consideration of each patient and will depend on the type and severity of the anaemia. The following points should be considered.

■ Observation

General observations of the patient should be made, such as colour of the skin, pallor, jaundice and any oedema or purpura which may be present. The patient's movements should be observed for any limb weakness, for example in pernicious anaemia, and also the degree of activity the patient is capable of without becoming tired or breathless.

■ Rest

Patients with severe anaemia may require complete bed rest and adequate sleep. Those who do not should be told of the importance of resting for periods and why they may be feeling weak and tired. Patients with anaemia are more susceptible to the development of pressure sores than they would otherwise be, so the avoidance of pressure by frequent changes of position is of utmost importance.

■ General hygiene and care of the skin

If very weak and severely anaemic the patient may initially have to be washed by the nurse. The nails should be kept clean and short; calamine lotion may be applied if pruritus is present. Mouth care is particularly important when soreness is present and mouthwashes should be offered frequently, possibly before and after a meal.

■ Eating and drinking

Meals should be light, easily digestible and well balanced, containing factors necessary for the normal development of red blood cells. The dietician may visit the patient as there may be particular difficulties associated with meals because of mouth soreness and dysphagia. Nutritious drinks may also be ordered to supplement the diet. Some drugs used for the treatment of anaemia, e.g. iron, may have to be administered in relation to mealtimes.

■ Elimination

Diarrhoea may be experienced as a result of some types of anaemia, and constipation may also develop as a result of some drug therapy, e.g. iron. Patients experiencing diarrhoea often need much reassurance due to embarrassment, particularly if bedpans are required frequently. The use of mild aperients may be necessary to overcome constipation. Specimens of faeces may have to be obtained for occult blood, and urine tested for urobilinogen, as well as 24-hour urine collections.

■ Drugs

Drugs should be administered as prescribed by the doctor. When a blood transfusion is in progress the patient must be closely observed (see p. 36) and, because of the dangers of overloading the circulation in a patient with severe anaemia, packed cells may be given. Antibiotic therapy may also be necessary in a patient with aplastic anaemia.

■ Maintenance of body temperature

An anaemic patient may require extra warmth as the oxygen necessary for the production of body heat may not be available in sufficient quantity.

■ Communication

Communication with the relatives should be continuous and monitored throughout the patient's stay. The need to take certain drugs for the rest of his life should be explained to both the patient and the relatives, as well as informing them of the possibility of crises occurring from time to time. The patient should be kept informed of all the investigations that may be necessary and should be adequately prepared.

■ LEUKAEMIA

Leukaemia is commonly known as cancer of the blood and describes abnormal proliferation of white cell tissue in the body, manifested by an increase in the total number of white blood cells, many of which are immature. The leukaemias are classified according to the white blood cell that is affected (see Table C, p. 46).

■ SUMMARY OF THE NURSING CARE FOR PATIENTS WITH LEUKAEMIA

A patient with acute or chronic leukaemia requires supportive, skilful nursing care. For two to three weeks after cytotoxic drug therapy there are very few normal white cells – as a result the patient is at increased risk of infection. He should be nursed in a single room, his attendants should be free from respiratory infections and septic skin lesions. Careful hand-washing on entering the room must be practised. It may be considered necessary for reverse barrier precautions to be observed.

■ Eating and drinking

A nutritious diet should be offered, high in calories and vitamins. Soreness of the mouth and the possible presence of ulcers should be considered and mouthwashes offered frequently. Diet may be

[*cont. p. 48*]

Table C Types of leukaemia:

	Acute leukaemia Myeloid Lymphatic Macrocytic
History	Onset is usually abrupt, frequently affects children
Causative factors if known	Unknown Possible overexposure to ionizing irradiation Possible virus Possible: some chemicals, e.g. benzol
Signs and symptoms	Fever and malaise Anaemia Bleeding manifestations, e.g. epistaxis; bleeding gums; purpura Mouth ulcers/sore throat Muscular and joint pains Enlargement of liver and spleen Enlargement of lymph nodes in acute lymphatic leukaemia
Specific investigations	Full blood count White cell count Differential white cell count Bleeding time Bone marrow puncture

Specific treatment	*Symptomatic and palliative*
	1 Short courses of chemotherapy:
	    a cytoxic drugs, e.g. vincristine sulphate
	    b immunosuppressants, e.g. corticosteroids
	    c antibiotics, e.g. actinomycin D
	    These courses may also be given intrathecally (blood/brain barrier)
	2 Blood transfusions (every 2–3 weeks)
	3 Platelet transfusions (daily)
	4 Radiotherapy: prophylactic to prevent 'cerebral leukaemia'
	5 Possible bone marrow transplantation in younger people: especially in myeloid variety when cytotoxic drugs are less effective

Prognosis	Fatal disease: death would occur within a few weeks but chemotherapy brings about remissions and extends life

Chronic myeloid leukaemia	Chronic lymphatic leukaemia
Onset is insidious (occurs mostly between the ages of 35–60 years) Affects both sexes equally	Onset is very insidious Commoner in males than females and between the ages of 45–75 years
Unknown Possibilities as for acute leukaemia	Unknown Possibilities as for other leukaemias
Vary from person to person Slow developing anaemia Loss of weight Spleen may be greatly enlarged Abdominal pain and tenderness of the spleen if infarction has occurred Bleeding manifestations	Very slow developing anaemia Presence of firm and painless lymph nodes in the body The spleen and liver may be enlarged There may or may not be bleeding manifestations Increased susceptibility to recurrent infections Haemolytic anaemia may develop
As for acute leukaemia	As for other leukaemias Paul-Bunnell test Biopsy of lymph node
Palliative symptomatic chemotherapy, e.g. busulphan. Radiotherapy of the spleen Blood transfusions Corticosteroids	Determined by the clinical state of the patient If treatment is necessary, radiotherapy to spleen Chemotherapy, e.g. chlorambucil Possible corticosteroids for haemolytic anaemia
Average duration of life is 2–3 years following diagnosis	Slowly progressive, death occurs within 5 years of diagnosis

supplemented by nutritious drinks, and fluids should be plentiful as the patient may be pyrexial. In the period immediately following treatment with cytotoxic drugs, only *cooked hot* food should be offered. This minimizes the risk of infection. The rapid destruction of white blood cells will also increase the level of uric acid in the blood which has to be eliminated by the kidneys. If the patient is unable to take oral fluids the doctor may set up an intravenous infusion to maintain adequate hydration. Fluid balance should be recorded.

In Table C examples of only some of the possible drugs that may be used for the treatment of leukaemia are given; it must be remembered that a *combination* of these drugs may be used and that they may be changed or administered at specific periods throughout the course of treatment. The aim of treatment is to suppress the development of excess abnormal white cells. Due to the side-effects that may be produced the patient is usually nursed in centres where there are adequate facilities for monitoring the patient's response to therapy.

■ Skin and general hygiene

Great care should be taken in the prevention of skin breakdown, by keeping the skin clean and free from perspiration, with frequent changing of the patient's position. Aids, such as sheepskins, a Ripple bed, may be considered necessary and should be selected appropriately for each patient. Careful handling of the patient should be exercised due to the increased tendency to bleed. The hair and nails should be kept clean and certain patients may wish to be helped with their make-up. Instructions relating to skin care when radiotherapy is being given should be carefully followed.

Particular attention should be paid to the mouth and the use of a soft-bristled toothbrush is appropriate. Measures should be taken to prevent the patient's lips from cracking.

■ Mobilization

The degree of mobility of which the patient is capable should be carefully assessed and the subsequent care should be planned to serve the patient's needs. Prevention of excessive pressure to certain areas must be maintained when the patient is sitting out in a chair. Adequate rest is important and provision should be made for this. Analgesics may be administered for pain.

■ Observation

Care of the patient should include observation of vital signs, reaction to drug therapy or radiotherapy, haemorrhage and signs of infection.

The nurse should be aware of the side-effects of certain drugs that may be used, so that the patient can be effectively observed for these. Depending on the drugs used these may include nausea, vomiting, diarrhoea, stomatitis, skin rash, alopecia. Many of the drugs cause bone marrow depression giving rise to anaemia, leucopaenia and thrombocytopaenia.

■ Elimination

Urinary output should be closely observed and recorded. Any diarrhoea which may occur as a result of chemotherapy should be reported.

Both urine and faeces may have to be tested for blood.

■ Communication

Communication with relatives should be maintained throughout the period of hospitalization and they should be kept fully informed concerning the patient's condition. Relatives may also want to be involved in the patient's care and should be allowed to do so as much as possible. Many patients will go home during periods of remission and the relatives may feel more confident about this if they have been allowed to participate in the patient's care at an earlier stage. In the case of children, parents should be given full support and should be allowed to stay with the child if they wish to; interest should also be shown towards other children in the family. Time should be allowed for talking to the family about their fears, in a suitable environment free from interruptions. The patient or the family may request a visit from the chaplain or their own minister and such requests should be granted.

Careful assessment of the needs of the patient and family will help determine where in the ward the patient will be best nursed. Due to the need to avoid exposure to infection, a single side-room may be most suitable and the reason why should be explained to the relatives. In the case of a child, when one or both parents are staying in the hospital, they should be told where the eating facilities and the toilets are. They should also be shown the location of telephones so that they can readily maintain contact with the rest of the family.

■ PRACTICE QUESTIONS

1 *What is meant by the following terms?*
  a Buffer systems.
  b Haematocrit.

  c Oxyhaemoglobin.
  d Erythropoiesis.
  e Erythropoietin.
  f Phagocytosis.
  g Diapedesis.
  h Histamine.
  i Immunoglobulins (antibodies).
  j Thromboplastin.
  k Prothrombin.
  l Agglutinogens.
  m Agglutinins.
  n ABO grouping system.
  o Rhesus factor.
  p Incompatible blood transfusion.
  q Anaemia.
  r Hypochlorhydria.
  s Plummer-Vinson syndrome.
  t Dysphagia.
  u Pernicious anaemia.
  v Macrocytic (cells).
  w Schilling test.
  x Thyroxine.
  y Aplastic anaemia.
  z Haemolytic anaemia.
  aa Thrombocytopenia.
  bb Leucopenia.
  cc Leucocytosis.

2 *Briefly explain the following:*
  a The function of red blood cells.
  b The function of white blood cells.
  c The functions of plasma proteins.
  d The mechanism of blood clotting.
  e Why blood group AB cannot be given to a patient whose blood is group A.
  f Why a patient with anaemia is hypoxic.
  g Why patients with rhesus negative blood should not receive blood which is rhesus positive.
  h Why patients with pernicious anaemia require intramuscular injections of vitamin B_{12} for the rest of their lives.
  i The development of jaundice in haemolytic anaemia.
  j Why a patient who has leukaemia may also have anaemia and a tendency to bleed.

3 *Mark the following statements true or false:*

  a Antimetabolites are drugs which interfere with chemical reactions within the leukaemia cells depriving them of essential factors.

  b Rhesus positive patients can receive blood which is rhesus positive or rhesus negative.

  c The iron from broken-down red blood cells is excreted in bile.

  d Neutrophils constitute the largest proportion of the granulocytes.

  e The monocytes are responsible for antibody formation.

  f Blood group A may be given to a patient who is blood group A B.

  g 42% of the population is blood group O.

  h Haemolytic anaemia is caused by excessive destruction of red blood cells.

  i Serum is similar to plasma without the clotting factors.

  j Agranulocytosis is the term used to describe an increase in the number of granular leucocytes.

■ **Answers**

1 *a* The presence and combination of certain substances and the physiological functions in the body which maintain the blood pH.

  b The volume of packed cells in a special calibrated tube. 45% of blood is made up of cells, i.e. the haematocrit.

  c Haemoglobin saturated with oxygen.

  d Formation of the red blood cells.

  e A hormone-like substance produced by the kidneys.

  f The process whereby cells are able to ingest foreign particles.

  g The movement of neutrophils through the capillary wall to the site of infection in the tissue.

  h A substance released in response to an antigen-antibody reaction. Antihistamine drugs oppose the action of histamine.

  i A substance produced by the body to destroy foreign substances (antigens). This is known as the antigen-antibody reaction.

  j Formed as a result of tissue damage or platelet breakdown and is necessary for the conversion of prothrombin into thrombin.

  k A substance made in the liver and vitamin K is necessary for its formation.

  l A substance carried in the red blood cells. They are described by the letters A and B.

  m Naturally occurring antibodies found in the plasma.

  n A system devised for identifying the main blood groups. A, B, AB and O, according to the presence of agglutinogens in the red blood cells or the absence of agglutinogens as in blood group O.

    o Another agglutinogen D discovered to be present in the red cells of about 85% of the population.

    p When the cells of blood transfused are destroyed by the agglutinins in the plasma, and is termed agglutination.

    q A deficiency in the quality and quantity of red blood cells accompanied by a reduction in the O_2 carrying substance haemoglobin.

    r A reduction in the production of hydrochloric acid.

    s Soreness of the mouth and tongue, atrophy of the papillae, dysphagia associated with iron deficiency anaemia.

    t Difficulty in swallowing.

    u The inability to absorb vitamin B_{12} due to the failure of the gastric mucosa to produce Castle's intrinsic factor.

    v Cells that are larger than usual.

    w A test performed to aid the diagnosis of vitamin B_{12} deficiency.

    x A hormone produced by the thyroid gland.

    y A decrease in the activity of the bone marrow giving rise to a reduction in the formation of red blood cells.

    z Anaemia caused through excessive destruction of red blood cells.

  aa A reduction in the formation of platelets.

  bb A reduction in the numbers of circulating white cells.

  cc An increase in the numbers of circulating white blood cells.

2 *a* To carry oxygen around the body on the haemoglobin.

    b Protect the body against infection; formation of immunoglobulins (antibodies); respond to allergic states; production of heparin and histamine.

    c Maintenance of blood viscosity and blood pH. Carriage of immunoglobulins and transportation of many substances. Provide blood clotting factors and assist with osmosis.

    d Damaged tissue and broken-down platelets are necessary for the formation of thromboplastin. This combines with prothrombin formed in the liver and converts it to thrombin for which calcium ions are also necessary. Thrombin then acts on the fibrinogen in plasma converting it into fibrin – a clot is then formed.

    e The agglutinins anti-B, present in the recipient's plasma, will destroy the agglutinogen B present in the donor's red blood, causing agglutination.

    f Hypoxia is the term used to describe a shortage of oxygen. In anaemia there is usually a shortage of haemoglobin to carry the oxygen.

    g Patients with rhesus negative blood do not have the agglutinogen D present in their red blood cells. Should they receive blood which is rhesus positive they will develop anti-D. This is of particular importance in young females and those of childbearing age.

h Due to the lack of Castle's intrinsic factor, they are unable to absorb any vitamin B_{12} taken orally, therefore adequate supplies have to be given by intramuscular injection.

i Excessive production of red blood cells results in excessive formation of the bile pigment bilirubin. Accumulation of this pigment in the blood gives rise to jaundice.

j Proliferation of leukaemic tissue causes an increase in the number of white cells. This abnormal increase interferes with the normal formation and 'crowding out' of the red blood cells and platelets. A reduction of the red cells will cause anaemia and a reduction of the platelets will give rise to a bleeding tendency.

3 *a* True
  b True
  c False
  d True
  e False
  f True
  g False
  h True
  i True
  j False

4 Respiration

The purpose of this section is to:
1 Outline the anatomy of the respiratory tract and lungs and the physiology of respiration.
2 Identify common diseases affecting respiration.
3 Describe the investigations and total management of the patient with diseases affecting respiration.

The respiratory system is associated with the exchange of gases between man and the environment. All body cells need a continuous supply of oxygen (O_2) and also need to be able to rid themselves of carbon dioxide (CO_2) which is produced by cell metabolism. As blood passes through the capillaries in the lungs it takes up oxygen from the alveoli and gives out carbon dioxide: this is external respiration. The blood transports the oxygen through the circulatory system and oxygen diffuses through the capillary walls into the body cells, the carbon dioxide produced diffuses from the body cells back into the capillaries for transportation: this is internal respiration.

The air inspired contains oxygen, carbon dioxide, nitrogen and water vapour and the temperature of this air varies. Expired air includes all of the above in different quantities and is at body temperature. The structure necessary to convey this air from the environment to the body includes:
a *The upper respiratory tract:*
nose
mouth
pharynx.
b *The lower respiratory tract:*
larynx
trachea
bronchi
lungs.

As the air passes through the nose, it is filtered, warmed and moistened by the ciliated columnar epithelium lining the nostrils and its rich blood supply. It then passes through the pharynx which is lined by mucous membrane. Food also passes through the oro- and laryngo-pharynx but is prevented from entering the larynx by a leaf-shaped structure called the epiglottis. Any particles of food that may find their way to the larynx will produce a violent cough due to a contraction of the pharyngeal muscle.

The larynx is a tube-like structure made up of muscles and a series of cartilages namely, the epiglottic, thyroid and cricoid cartilages and a pair of arytenoid cartilages. It contains the vocal chords necessary for the production of voice sounds and is continuous with the pharynx above and with the trachea below. The trachea is a fibro-elastic tube supported by incomplete rings of cartilage to prevent collapse of the tube; it is lined by ciliated epithelium.

The trachea divides at the level of the sternal angle into the right and left branches or bronchi (Fig. 3). The main bronchi divide further into several bronchi like the branches of a tree and the farther away these tubes go from the main bronchus the smaller they become, forming bronchioles. They contain cartilage and much smooth muscle. The bronchioles lead into air sacs through ducts called the alveolar sacs which are thin-walled structures containing air and capillaries. It is here that the exchange of gases takes place. The bronchi, and the bronchioles are contained in the lungs, which are two large spongy organs contained in the thoracic cavity. The lungs are enveloped in a serous membrane called the pleura. The pleura that covers the surface of the lung is called the visceral pleura and, as it is a closed sac, it is continuous with the parietal pleura which lines the wall of the thoracic cavity. Between the visceral and parietal pleura is a potential space. The

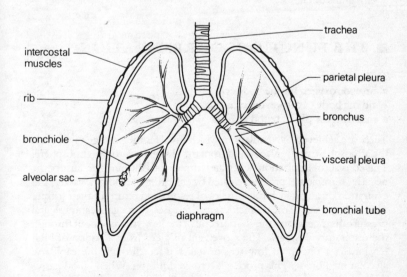

Fig. 3 Structures necessary for respiration

thoracic cavity is formed by the thoracic vertebrae posteriorly, the sternum anteriorly, and is surrounded by 12 pairs of ribs providing good protection for its contents. The blood supply to the lungs is provided by the bronchial arteries; the pulmonary artery also conveys blood to the lungs for oxygenation; blood is collected by veins and returned to the left side of the heart by the pulmonary veins. These vessels enter and leave the lungs at the hilum.

Each lung is made up of lobes, the right lung having three lobes and the left lung having two. Each lobe is further divided into segments according to the specific bronchus that supplies the segment (broncho-pulmonary segment).

Muscles of respiration are:
a diaphragm
b intercostal muscles.
Accessory muscles of respiration include:
a pectoralis major
b serratus anterior
c sternomastoid
d anterior abdominals
e latissimus dorsi.

■ THE FUNCTIONS OF RESPIRATION

These are to:
a provide oxygen for the body cells
b rid the body of carbon dioxide
c maintain the pH of blood at 7.4.

These are achieved by ventilation, which involves the passage of air from the atmosphere to the alveoli and from the alveoli back to the atmosphere. This consists of inspiration, when air is drawn into the lungs because of the negative intrapleural pressure created by enlarging the thoracic cavity, and expiration during which the muscles of respiration return to their former positions, the size of the thoracic cavity decreases, the negative intrapleural pressure disappears and the elastic recoil of the lungs drives air out through the respiratory passages. The movement of gases from a region of high tension to a region of low tension takes place through the capillary/alveolar membrane. This process is termed diffusion. When blood passes through the lung capillaries the tension (partial pressure) of oxygen in the alveoli is higher than that of the blood, and it passes through the membrane to a region of lower tension. The tension of carbon dioxide as it passes through the lungs is greater in the blood than in the alveolar air, and so passes through the membrane to the region of low tension. The same principle applies at tissue level. Diffusion may be affected if changes occur in the alveolar membrane as a result of disease and/or if there is alteration in the flow of blood through the lung capillaries. The ventilation/perfusion ratio must be correct for effective diffusion.

Respiration is under the control of the respiratory centre in the medulla of the brain, which in turn is influenced by the pH and the carbon dioxide level in the blood. The respiratory centre is stimulated to increase the rate and depth of breathing by an increase in the carbon dioxide level.

Inspiration is cut short by the presence of stretch receptors in the lung which are stimulated by the expansion of the lung tissue. These receptors send sensory impulses via the vagus nerve to the respiratory centre.

Respiration is modified by the effects of the higher centres on the respiratory centre during the acts of talking, singing and swallowing.

The lungs are in the thoracic cavity which acts as an airtight box. There is no space between the inside of the thorax and the outside of the lung. The two sides of the chest are separated by the mediastinum which contains the heart and great vessels, the oesophagus, trachea, thoracic duct and the thymus gland. Should air enter this airtight box from a chest wound, for example, or from a ruptured bulla, air is drawn in between the pleural layers, the potential space then becomes a real one, the lung collapses and ventilation is inadequate.

The presence of air in the pleural cavity is called a pneumothorax. The presence of clear fluid in the pleural cavity is called a pleural effusion (hydrothorax). Pus in the pleural cavity is referred to as empyema. Blood in the pleural cavity is referred to as haemothorax. A collapsed lung causes a mediastinal shift.

Of the 500ml of air taken in during normal quiet inspiration, only 350ml will reach the lungs, because 150ml remains in the air passages; in expired air following inspiration the first 150ml of this will be dead space air, as it has been no farther than the air passages and is not involved in the exchange of gases. The volume of dead space is therefore 150ml.

□ *Definitions*

Tidal volume: The volume of air inspired or expired with each respiration during normal quiet breathing – approximately 500ml.

Inspiratory capacity: Maximum amount of air that can be inspired with effort – approximately 3400ml.

Inspiratory reserve volume: The volume of inspired air in excess of the tidal volume – approximately 3000ml.

Expiratory reserve volume: The volume of air that can be forcibly expired following a normal quiet expiration – approximately 1100ml.

Residual volume: The volume of air remaining in the lungs following a forced expiration – approximately 1200ml.

Vital capacity: the maximum volume of air which can be expired following an inspiration of maximum capacity – 4000 to 5000ml. It is the sum of the inspiratory and expiratory reserve volumes plus the tidal volume.

Total lung capacity: The vital capacity plus the residual volume constitutes the total lung capacity – 5200–6000ml.

■ COMMON CONDITIONS AFFECTING THE RESPIRATORY SYSTEM

These are:

1 Bronchitis: acute, chronic
2 Emphysema
3 Asthma
4 Pneumonia
5 Carcinoma of the lung
6 Cor pulmonale
7 Pulmonary embolism.

■ Bronchitis

□ *Acute*

This is an acute inflammation of the trachea and the bronchial tubes and frequently follows an upper respiratory tract infection and influenza. Factors which may predispose to the development of an infection include a dusty, damp and foggy atmosphere, and smoking. The severity of the disease varies and the development of pneumonia as a complication is a possibility. Initially the patient may complain of pain or discomfort behind the sternum accompanied by a dry irritating cough. As the infection spreads the patient becomes pyrexial with a productive cough, the sputum being mucopurulent. Due to the irritation the bronchioles may go into spasm producing difficulty in breathing and wheezing respirations. A specimen of sputum may be obtained for culture and sensitivity. The doctor may prescribe/advise any of the following:

  i Antibiotic therapy.
 ii Bronchodilator – if bronchospasm is present.
iii Oxygen therapy.
 iv Sedative linctus, if cough is disturbing sleep.

v Bed rest.
vi Steam inhalations.
vii High fluid intake.
viii Chest physiotherapy.

■ **Chronic bronchitis and emphysema**

These two diseases often occur together and are referred to as chronic obstructive airway disease. Chronic bronchitis develops as a result of being exposed for prolonged periods to irritation, which may be caused by tobacco smoke (particularly cigarettes), atmospheric pollution, and exposure to dust, smoke and fumes; the condition itself may be further provoked by a damp, foggy climate. It is commoner in males than females and there may be a heredity factor involved.

The bronchial mucosa undergoes changes with swelling of the mucous membrane and enlargement of the goblet and mucus-secreting cells, which are overactive and produce large amounts of mucus which suffices to plug the smaller bronchioles and affect ventilation. Eventually, due to obstruction to the airway, which is greater during expiration, air becomes trapped in the alveoli which causes overdistension and possible rupture. Infection superimposed on this leads to further tissue damage. This damage and overdistension of the alveoli is termed emphysema. There now develops an imbalance in the ventilation, i.e. in the perfusion ratio. Chronic bronchitis is a disease which usually progresses over a number of years. The patient may start developing coughs during cold, damp winter months until, eventually, the cough becomes permanent. Dyspnoea and wheezing are progressive with the production of tenacious white or mucopurulent sputum, and over a period of time the patient may develop symptoms of hypoxia and hypercapnia. The course of the disease varies considerably. The doctor may order the following investigations:

i Radiological examination of the chest.
ii Full blood counts, and differential white cell count.
iii Specimens of sputum for culture and sensitivity, acid fast bacilli and cytological examination.
iv Lung function tests.
v Possibly a bronchoscopy/bronchogram.
vi Analysis of blood gases.
vii ECG.

□ *Treatment*
The treatment ordered may be treatment and control of the infection by antibiotic therapy. The patient should be advised to seek medical advice at the first sign of a respiratory infection. He should also be advised to give up

smoking and, occasionally, it may be necessary for the patient to change his occupation and/or even live in a different area.

Maintenance of ventilation may be obtained by humidification of room air, adequate fluid intake, physiotherapy to promote expectoration, breathing exercises and postural drainage. Oxygen therapy may be prescribed but must be administered with care. The concentration of oxygen is usually prescribed, as well as the rate of flow, as some patients with chronic respiratory disease become accustomed to a higher pCO_2 and the respiratory centre is stimulated by the hypoxia. The administration of excess oxygen could, therefore, cause depression of respirations. A bronchodilator may also be prescribed if bronchospasm is present. The appropriate medication may also be prescribed for a troublesome cough. The obese patient is advised to lose weight.

■ Asthma

Asthma is narrowing of the bronchi due to spasm of the surrounding smooth muscle and swelling of the mucous membrane accompanied by viscid secretions. The narrowing of the bronchi causes inadequate ventilation which is more marked on expiration, resulting in air being trapped in the alveoli causing distension. As asthma is episodic it tends to occur suddenly at any time. The patient presents with dyspnoea, particularly on expiration, accompanied by wheezing. Expiration is a conscious effort, bringing into play the accessory muscles of respiration which can prove exhausting for the patient. Asthma most commonly begins in childhood or middle age, but can start at any age.

Asthma may be caused by hypersensitivity (allergy) to certain drugs, foods or, more commonly, to substances inhaled. Heredity appears to be another factor in the development of asthma and patients often give a family history of allergic conditions such as eczema or hay fever. Asthmatic reactions may develop as a response to frequent respiratory infections. Any factor which causes irritation of the bronchi such as tobacco smoke, infection, dust, etc., may provoke an attack of asthma as well as causing emotional stress.

An attack of asthma may end abruptly but if the attack persists for many hours or, possibly, days the term severe acute asthma (status asthmaticus) is used. It is sometimes possible to desensitize a patient if, following sensitivity tests, a specific allergen can be identified. A child with severe asthma may develop a 'pigeon chest' deformity.

Treatment of an asthmatic attack will depend on its severity and the condition of the patient. The doctor may require a chest radiograph, full blood count and differential white cell count, and the number of eosinophils is usually increased. Analysis of sputum, blood gases and pH may also be required, as well as lung function tests.

◻ *Treatment*

The treatment may include the prescription of oxygen therapy and drugs to relieve bronchial spasm, e.g. ephedrine, aminophylline, salbutamol, orciprenaline or, possibly, adrenaline. The drugs are administered by the route prescribed by the doctor; some may be given subcutaneously, intravenously, orally, by rectal suppository or inhalation. Salbutamol and orciprenaline can be given by inhalation from pressurized dispensers or nebulizers. The administration of a corticosteroid drug is sometimes considered necessary. An antibiotic may be prescribed if an infection is present, and dehydration may require intravenous replacements of fluid.

When the attack of asthma is controlled, the patient and relatives are usually advised what precautions to take in preventing attacks. Discussions may be necessary if emotional stress is a causative factor, to determine how these effects can be minimized where possible.

■ **Pneumonia**

This is inflammation of the lung. There are different kinds of pneumonia and the type is usually used to specify the pneumonia present. If the pneumonia is caused by a bacteria or virus then it is usually referred to by the specific causative organism, e.g. pneumococcal pneumonia or staphylococcal pneumonia as the case may be. Pneumonia may also be referred to according to the anatomical distribution of the disease, e.g. lobar pneumonia or segmental pneumonia if confined to a lobe or segment, but if the distribution is widespread it is referred to as broncho-pneumonia or lobular pneumonia. Pneumonia may also develop as a result of existing disease of the respiratory tract, it may be caused by the inhalation of vomitus (aspiration pneumonia), or it may be due to physical weakness and immobilization in bed (hypostatic pneumonia).

Pneumonia most commonly occurs during the winter months and all age-groups are susceptible. The manifestations of pneumonia vary with the type. Those types caused by organisms are usually sudden in outset with an abrupt rise in temperature, shivering and possibly rigor. The pulse and respiratory rates increase. A cough may be present which is initially painful and unproductive, but which gradually becomes less painful and productive. The patient may also complain of pain on respiration (pleuritic pain) and in pneumococcal pneumonia the sputum is often rust-coloured. Other symptoms may include headache and neck stiffness. Herpes simplex may be present around the nose and mouth and cyanosis may be present.

Inflammatory exudate develops in the alveoli and areas of the lung tissue become consolidated; ventilation and diffusion are usually affected, with a reduction in the oxygen tension of the blood.

Treatment of pneumonia usually involves modified bed rest until the temperature returns to normal. The doctor usually prescribes the appropriate antibiotic therapy, analgesia for pain, and a linctus preparation for a troublesome unproductive cough. Oxygen is administered as prescribed and breathing exercises taught by the physiotherapist. Prior to this treatment the doctor may order some or all of the following investigations:

a Specimen of sputum for culture and sensitivity.
b Blood for full blood count, differential white cell count, estimation of electrolytes, analysis of blood gases and pH.
c Chest radiograph.

Should the patient not respond to treatment or complications develop, further treatment may be necessary, involving chest aspiration for pleural effusion. Delayed resolution may require bronchoscopy and bronchogram, inhalations and postural drainage.

■ Carcinoma of the lung

The incidence of lung carcinoma is greater in males than females and cigarette smoking is considered to be an important causative factor, as well as atmospheric pollution and exposure to dusts and chemical gases. The types of tumours frequently found are those giving rise to oat cell carcinoma, squamous carcinoma and adenocarcinoma.

The symptoms develop according to the location of the tumour, and sometimes the tumour is found during the course of a routine chest radiological examination without the patient's having manifested any symptoms. Sometimes the patient may present with symptoms of complications, such as pneumonia, obstruction of a bronchus, lung abscess, pleural effusion, and symptoms which arise from pressure being exerted on other structures in the mediastinum. Some tumours are found to produce secretions similar to those produced by glands of the endocrine system. Symptoms may include a cough with haemoptysis, and possibly mucopurulent sputum with progressive bronchial obstruction giving rise to atelectasis. Dyspnoea and a persistent wheeze may be experienced as well as pain in the chest. The patient may complain of tiredness and loss of weight with the development of anaemia.

Investigations may include:
a Sputum for cytological examination.
b Chest radiograph.
c Bronchoscopy and biopsy.

Treatment may be surgical removal of the lobe or of the lung (pneumonectomy), radiotherapy, cytotoxic drugs. Early recognition and treatment of the disease is significant in terms of prognosis.

■ Cor pulmonale

This is a cardiovascular disease which develops secondary to disease of the lungs, commonly occurring with chronic bronchitis and emphysema. The cardiovascular changes occur as a result of the respiratory failure, causing abnormal levels of blood gases and an imbalance in the ventilation/perfusion ratio. The aim of treatment is to improve and maintain alveolar ventilation.

■ Pulmonary embolism

This commonly arises from a deep vein thrombosis, and if the embolism is large it may cause sudden death; otherwise patients complain of a sudden tightness or pain in the chest, difficulty in breathing and a sudden need to have their bowels opened. They may be cyanosed, pale and sweaty, with a rapid thready pulse and a low blood pressure.

The *treatment* usually involves lying the patient flat with one or two pillows, administering oxygen and analgesics for pain, and commencing anticoagulant therapy, controlled by estimation of the prothrombin time.

■ SUMMARY OF THE NURSING CARE FOR PATIENTS WITH RESPIRATORY DISEASES

A patient admitted to hospital with a respiratory condition frequently requires close observation and should be placed in a position in the ward where this is best achieved. The fact that the patient has difficulty in breathing is in itself a frightening experience and much reassurance is required. All equipment that may be necessary should be regularly and frequently checked for its working order, including oxygen and suction apparatus and humidifiers.

■ Mobility

Initially the patient will be placed in bed or, in some instances, a chair may be found to be more suitable. Due to the difficulty experienced in breathing, the patient may quickly become exhausted. Often the patient may be allowed to assume the position in which he is most comfortable, which is sitting up, possibly leaning forward on a bed table on which a pillow has been placed. In this sitting up position the patient finds it easier to breathe as the thoracic cavity can expand without too much restriction. Adequate pillows are necessary to support the patient, including the patient's head, and the bedclothes over the patient should be loose and unrestrictive. Cot sides may be considered necessary if the patient is drowsy. The patient should have his position changed frequently by the nurses to prevent the development of pressure sores. As his condition improves, mobilization is increased and in some conditions, e.g. chronic bronchitis, the patient's degree of mobility is assessed and recorded.

■ Observations

These are made at regular intervals and as frequently as the patient's condition warrants. Observations include temperature and pulse rate, the rate and depth of respirations and movement of the two sides of the chest; any abnormal sounds produced by respiration should be noted. The presence and degree of cyanosis should be observed and undue restlessness and confusion should be reported to the doctor as this could be indicative of hypoxia. Observation should be made of the amount and colour of sputum and it is important that there is adequate provision of containers with covers.

■ Oxygen therapy

All the necessary precautions should be taken during the administration of oxygen to ensure the safety of the patient and other persons in the environment. Adequate humidification should be available because of the drying effects of oxygen on the respiratory mucosa and the correct appliance should be used for its administration. Oxygen is prescribed by the doctor and for some conditions it is important that the correct concentration of oxygen is given as well as the rate of flow. If masks or nasal cannulae are being used the nurse should ensure that adequate lengths of tubing are available and that the masks fit comfortably on the face.

■ Physiotherapy

Deep breathing and postural exercises are frequently necessary. To facilitate the removal of secretions, postural drainage may be employed. This means that the patient is placed in a position, depending on which lung segment requires drainage, so that mucus will drain from the periphery to the larger bronchi and trachea. Here the mucus may be more readily aspirated by the use of a suction apparatus or expectorated by coughing. Preparations may be used to promote expectoration in the form of oral medication (expectorant). Liquefication of secretions may also be achieved by the use of local aerosol preparations (mucolytic agents). If the patient is experiencing pain when coughing, support over the painful area may be required. Movement of secretions is also achieved by frequent changes of positon.

■ Eating and drinking

Small frequent meals are more suitable for patients who are having difficulty in breathing and assistance with feeding may be required. An increased fluid intake is necessary (unless there are contra-indications for this) to help liquefy the bronchial secretions and, if the patient is pyrexial, as in pneumonia or acute bronchitis for example, to prevent dehydration. If the patient's appetite is poor, nutritonal drinks may be given to supplement the diet. Care of any infusions should be maintained if fluids are administered intravenously. A record of the fluid balance is maintained.

■ Skin and general hygiene

Care should be taken to maintain the skin in good condition. Assistance may be needed with washing when the patient is dyspnoeic and acutely ill. Frequent washes are required when the patient is pyrexial, with frequent change of bed linen and nightwear. A fan may be used to help keep the patient cool. The presence of herpes simplex associated with pneumonia should be noted.

Facilities for cleaning the teeth and mouthwashes should be offered frequently due to the drying effects of oxygen therapy and fever, and the expectoration of infected sputum. The fingernails and toenails should be kept clean and short and any clubbing of the fingers which may develop with some chronic respiratory diseases should be noted.

■ Elimination

All urinary output should be noted. Constipation causes abdominal distension which will cause further respiratory difficulties and should be avoided. Mild aperients may be required. The use of a commode may prove less of a strain to the patient than using a bedpan.

■ Sputum

The patient should be provided with adequate tissues and a sputum carton with a lid for the purposes of expectoration. The cartons should be renewed as often as is necessary and should be kept within easy reach of the patient, as well as a bag for the disposal of used tissues. All sputum should be carefully handled and correctly disposed of. Organisms may spread from one person to another by droplet infection and in some instances the patient may require barrier nursing. It should be explained to the relatives why this is necessary.

■ Administration of drugs

All drugs are administered as prescribed and the patient is observed for their effects. Analgesia and suitable sedation may be prescribed. Opiates should be avoided because of their tendency to depress the respiratory centre.

■ Communication

Communication is maintained at all times with the patient's relatives and guidance, advice and support is given where necessary. In some instances the patient's whole way of life may require adaptation. In other cases the family may need advice about keeping rooms free of possible irritants, as in asthma. Furniture, floors and walls may require frequent damp-dusting and flowers, carpets and curtains may need to be kept free of dust. The patient may be forced to change his occupation and the help of a medical social worker and the disablement resettlement officer (DRO) may be required. Close communication should be maintained with the community and social services in relation to home adaptations and the continued provision of oxygen therapy and medication at home under supervision.

■ PRACTICE QUESTIONS

1 *What is meant by the following terms:*
   a Inspiration.
   b Expiration.
   c Mediastinum.
   d Pneumothorax.
   e Haemothorax.
   f Pleural effusion.
   g Empyema.
   h Emphysema.
   i Tidal volume.

j Acute bronchitis.

k Dyspnoea.

l Bronchogram.

m Asthma.

n Allergy.

o Haemoptysis.

p Bronchopneumonia.

q Postural drainage.

r Expectorant.

s Respiratory centre.

t Oxygen.

2 *Briefly explain the following:*

a The function of respiration.

b Why food does not enter the air passages during swallowing.

c The process of ventilation.

d The passage of oxygen from the alveolar air sacs to the blood capillaries.

e The changes which take place in the air passages and lungs in chronic bronchitis.

f The condition of hypercapnia.

g Why the concentration of oxygen may be prescribed when patients have chronic lung disease.

h The effects of a bronchodilator drug.

i The reasons for aspirating fluid from the pleural cavity.

j What is a cough?

3 *Mark the following statements true or false:*

a The respiratory tissues receive their nourishment via the pulmonary artery.

b The rate of respiration varies with age.

c Narcotics and barbiturates are examples of drugs that reduce respiratory activity.

d Apnoea is the term used to describe a decrease in the respiratory rate.

e The number of eosinophils is increased in allergic states, such as asthma.

f Perfusion refers to the movement of oxygen and carbon dioxide between the blood capillaries and body cells.

g Chronic bronchitis, emphysema and asthma are classified as chronic obstructive airways diseases.

h Empyema may be a complication of pneumonia.

i Pneumoconiosis is a term used for dust diseases of the lungs.

j Respiration is controlled by the respiratory centre in the medulla.

■ **Answers**

1 *a* The activity of air being drawn into the lungs.
  b The activity of air being expelled from the lungs.
  c The area in the thoracic cavity not taken up by the lungs but containing the heart, great blood vessels, oesophagus, trachea and thymus gland.
  d Air in the pleural cavity.
  e Blood in the pleural cavity.
  f Fluid in the pleural cavity.
  g Pus in the pleural cavity.
  h Thinning and distension of the alveolar air sacs.
  i The volume of air breathed in or out during normal quiet respirations – approximately 500ml.
  j Acute inflammation of the trachea and bronchi which may complicate an upper respiratory tract infection.
  k Difficulty in breathing.
  l A special radiological examination of the bronchial tree following the insertion of a radio-opaque substance to outline the bronchial tubes.
  m Spasm of the smooth muscle of the bronchioles accompanied by swelling of the mucous membrane causing narrowing of the tubes.
  n Hypersensitivity to certain substances.
  o The term used to describe the coughing-up of blood in the sputum.
  p Also called lobular pneumonia when the distribution of the disease is widespread.
  q Adopting the appropriate position which will facilitate the movement of fluid and mucus from the periphery of the lungs towards the larger bronchi and trachea where they are more readily coughed up.
  r Drugs that liquefy and increase secretions.
  s A collection of nerve cells found in the medulla of the brain which control respiration.
  t A colourless, odourless gas that is essential for normal cell metabolism.

2 *a* To provide oxygen for the body cells and to rid the body of carbon dioxide. Also maintains the pH of blood at 7.4.
  b The presence of food stimulates the muscles of the pharynx to contract, directing food and fluid into the oesophagus, and closing off the entrance to the nose. The larynx is closed off by the epiglottis.
  c The movement of air in and out of the lungs achieved by varying the size of the thoracic cavity and elasticity of lung tissue.
  d Oxygen moves from a region of high tension to low, by the process of diffusion through the capillary wall. When blood (having given off

oxygen to the tissues) returns to the lung capillaries, the partial pressure of oxygen in the alveoli is higher than that of the blood. Oxygen then diffuses through the membrane into the blood to a region of lower tension.

e Swelling of mucous membrane. Enlargement of goblet and mucus secreting cells. Destruction of cilia. Eventual thinning and over-distension of the alveoli. Superimposed infection may lead to further tissue damage.

f A state where there is too much carbon dioxide in the blood.

g Due to chronic lung disease the respiratory centre has become accustomed to increased amounts of carbon dioxide and is rather stimulated by the hypoxia. Therefore if high concentrations of oxygen are administered the respiratory centre may be depressed.

h Dilating the bronchial tissue by causing relaxation of the smooth muscles.

i *Diagnostic purposes*: To establish whether fluid is purulent or serous. To detect presence of carcinoma cells. To isolate organism.
Treatment: To remove excessive fluid. To drain purulent effusion.

j A protective reflex. It occurs in response to irritation. Stimulus may arise in the respiratory tract (fluid, secretions, tumours, inflammation, dust, particles, foreign bodies, very hot or very cold air). Stimuli from outside due to pressure being exerted on the respiratory tract (inflammation of pleura, tumours in the oesophagus, aortic aneurysm, large mediastinal lymph nodes).

3 *a* False
  b True
  c True
  d False
  e True
  f False
  g False
  h True
  i True
  j True

5 The kidneys

The purpose of this chapter is:
1 To indicate the structure and function of the kidneys.
2 To identify the investigations and common conditions affecting the kidneys.
3 To describe the total care and management of patients with diseases of the kidneys.

■ THE FUNCTIONS OF THE KIDNEYS

These are to:
  i maintain the fluid and electrolyte balance
 ii excrete waste products of metabolism
iii maintain the blood pH at a constant level.

The kidneys are situated in the posterior abdomen behind the peritoneal cavity, at the level of the first lumbar vertebra. The right kidney is slightly lower than the left due to the presence of the liver on the right side. The two kidneys are encapsulated by a fibrous capsule surrounded by the peri-renal fat. The suprarenal (adrenal) glands are situated on the upper pole of each kidney. Urine is formed by the functioning unit of the kidney, the nephron, and is conveyed to the bladder by the ureters which leave the kidneys at the pelvis (of the kidney). Urine is conveyed from the bladder to the exterior by means of the urethra.

The blood supply to the kidneys is via the renal artery and drainage is through the renal vein.

Urine is formed by the nephrons, of which there are approximately one million in each kidney. The nephron is a tubular microscopic structure lined by specialized tubular cells (Fig. 4).

The supply of blood to the kidneys is important in relation to the formation of urine. They receive a good supply, about a quarter of the cardiac output (1200ml) every minute. After entering the kidney the renal artery branches into smaller arterioles and the afferent arterioles supply the glomeruli (tufts of capillaries), which are found in Bowman's capsule of the nephron. As the blood passes through the glomerulus it passes into the efferent arterioles, forming a capillary network surrounding the tubules. This then drains into the venous system and, eventually, into the inferior vena cava.

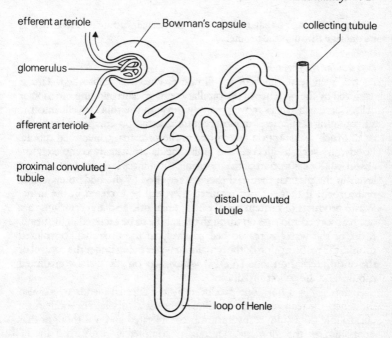

Fig. 4 A nephron

■ The processes involved in the formation of urine

  i Glomerular filtration.
 ii Tubular reabsorption.
iii Tubular secretion.

□ *Glomerular filtration*

The pressure of blood in the glomerular capillaries (70mmHg) is higher than in the other capillaries of the body. Deducted from this is the osmotic pressure of the plasma proteins (25mmHg) and the hydrostatic pressure in Bowman's capsule (10mmHg), giving a net filtration pressure of 35mmHg. The substances which pass through the walls of the capillary into the tubule are determined by their size. Those generally not filtered are the plasma proteins and the blood cells. One tenth of the blood passing through the glomerulus every minute is filtered, and the fluid formed in the tubule at this point is called the glomerular filtrate – thus the glomerular filtration rate is approximately 120ml of water per minute. However, the average urinary output in 24 hours is approximately 1500ml

(1ml per minute) so that 119ml of the glomerular filtrate is reabsorbed in its passage through the tubule.

□ *Tubular reabsorption*

As has been seen, much of the filtrate produced is reabsorbed. This is achieved by the presence of the capillary network surrounding the tubular cells. Some substances move passively through the tubular cells into the surrounding capillaries, but most require an active process provided by the cells. Much reabsorption takes place in the proximal convoluted tubule. Foodstuffs such as glucose and amino acids are usually completely re-absorbed. Reabsorption of the inorganic substances is dependent on their levels in the plasma; that is, if they are required by the body they will be reabsorbed; if they are not required they will be excreted in the urine. Waste products of protein metabolism, urea, uric acid and creatinine are not reabsorbed and pass on through the tubule to be excreted in the urine. Most of the water is reabsorbed passively in the proximal convoluted tubule, the reabsorption of the remaining water being under the control of the antidiuretic hormone (ADH) which acts on the distal convoluted tubules and the collecting tubules.

Aldosterone is a hormone produced by the adrenal glands which also influences the reabsorption of sodium in the distal tubule. The mechanism controlling potassium reabsorption is complicated and it is thought that potassium in the glomerular filtrate is completely reabsorbed in the proximal tubule, any excess being secreted into the tubule in the distal portion.

□ *Tubular secretion*

The tubular cells have the ability to secrete certain substances into the glomerular filtrate. Some toxic substances, drugs and excess acids and alkalis are removed from the body by tubular secretion, thus maintaining the blood pH at 7.4.

It is believed that the urine is concentrated in the collecting tubules and that water is extracted from them by osmosis as the tubule passes through tissues of varying osmolarity.

■ **Urine**

Urine is a fluid of varying shades of yellow. It has a specific gravity (concentration of solutes in the urine) of 1.012 to 1.025 and fresh urine is usually acid in reaction. It contains water (90–95%); waste products of protein metabolism, i.e. urea, uric acid and creatinine; inorganic salts and the pigment urochrome.

□ *Some abnormal constituents*
  Blood
  Pus
  Casts
  Glucose
  Plasma proteins (albumin)
  Ketone bodies

□ *Definitions*
Haematuria: blood in the urine.
Oliguria: decrease in urine production.
Anuria: complete cessation of urinary flow.
Polyuria: a considerble increase in the volume of urea.
Nocturia: emptying of the bladder during the night.
Dysuria: painful micturition.

  Micturition is both a voluntary and an involuntary process and is stimulated by the volume of urine in the bladder affecting the stretch receptors present.

  All patients admitted to hospital have their urine routinely tested for the presence of abnormal constituents, as well as note being made of the volume, appearance, reaction and specific gravity.

Erythropoietin and renin are both substances produced by the kidney. The former is necessary for the formation of red blood cells and the latter acts on plasma protein to form angiotensin which is a powerful vasoconstrictor.

■ DISEASES OF THE KIDNEYS

■ Acute glomerulonephritis

This often develops a few weeks following a sore throat or respiratory infection due to haemolytic streptococci. The organism has not been isolated in the kidneys or urine and it is thought that nephritis is an antigen/antibody reaction following the infection. The glomeruli of the kidneys undergo inflammatory changes. The condition can occur at any age but most commonly affects children and adolescents.

  The onset is usually sudden with a reduced urinary output, haematuria and the development of oedema, initially of the face. The patient may complain of pain and tenderness in the loins and a headache. There may also be pyrexia, loss of appetite, nausea, vomiting and hypertension.

  Complications include cerebral and pulmonary oedema, uraemia and cardiac failure.

◻ *Specific investigations*

a Examination of the blood – erythrocyte sedimentation rate (ESR)
                            – antistreptolysin O titre
                            – urea and electrolyte levels
b Nasal and throat swabs for culture and sensitivity.
c Urine specimen for microscopy.
d Renal function tests.

◻ *Treatment*

The patient must rest and should be confined to bed for a length of time that will vary from one patient to another. This is usually until the patient feels well and his temperature has subsided, as some of the abnormalities in the urine may remain for several months.

◻ *Diet and fluid regulation*

Fluids are usually restricted to 500ml a day, plus the equivalent of the previous day's output. Frequent and regular estimations of the urea and electrolytes are made. Diet consists mainly of carbohydrates and fats with restriction of protein. Salt is restricted, depending on the severity of the oedema. As diuresis occurs and the hypertension and haematuria subside, protein is gradually increased in the diet as a preliminary to a normal diet being resumed.

   Antibiotic therapy is commenced to eradicate the haemolytic streptococcal infection. If the patient does not respond, peritoneal dialysis or haemodialysis may be necessary. 90% of children who develop acute glomerulonephritis make a complete recovery. In some patients signs and symptoms may persist and they may pass through a subacute phase to develop chronic glomerulonephritis; others may develop renal failure.

◻ *Specific observations*

Temperature, pulse and respiration taken at regular intervals until temperature subsides. Blood pressure is taken daily or more frequently if requested by the doctor.
Fluid balance: all fluids administered to the patient and all urine passed should be accurately measured and recorded. Daily testing of urine for protein.

■ Chronic glomerulonephritis

This is a disease which may develop as a result of acute glomerulonephritis, or there may be no history of a previous disease, the chronic glomerulonephritis having slowly developed over a number of years. Changes gradually take place in the kidney tissue, resulting in destruction of the functioning units (nephrons); the course and progress of the disease varies considerably from patient to patient. The manifestations of the disease depend on the stage at which the patient presents. Eventually the patient will complain of symptoms arising from the inability of the kidneys to maintain their function. There will be signs of fluid and electrolyte imbalance as well as acidosis.

The management of the patient is based on the stage of the disease and is regulated by dietary and fluid intake, based on the laboratory results of tests made on the urine and blood. If the kidneys cannot adequately get rid of waste products, even when the intake of protein and fluids are regulated in the diet, dialysis may be considered.

■ Pyelonephritis (acute)

This is inflammation of the kidney substance as well as the pelvis (renal), most commonly caused by the Escherichia bacillus (*E coli*) normally present in the colon. It is occasionally caused by staphylococci or streptococci. It is commoner in women than men and this may be due to the anatomic relation of the female urethra to the rectum. Predisposing factors include obstruction to the flow of urine caused by calculi or strictures, tumours or congenital malformation; enlarged prostate gland and stasis of urine in the bladder may cause reflux of urine into the ureter.

During pregnancy stasis of urine is associated with an enlarged uterus and the effects of progesterone on the ureters. The importance of maintaining the highest standards of asepsis during the procedure of catheterization cannot be over-emphasized in relation to preventing the introduction of organisms into the urinary tract.

The onset of the condition is usually sudden with a pyrexia, nausea and vomiting; the patient complains of pain and tenderness in the loin, possibly radiating to the iliac fossa and the groins. There may be pain or burning sensation on micturition and the urine is usually cloudy.

□ *Specific investigations*
a Midstream specimen of urine (MSU) for culture and sensitivity.
b Urine for microscopy.
c Blood for full blood count (leucocytosis usually present).
Management of the patient includes bed rest and an increased fluid intake. Appropriate measures should be taken to keep the pyrexial patient comfortable, with frequent refreshing washes, an electric fan and changes of bed linen and nightwear. The doctor will prescribe the appropriate antibiotic or sulphonamide therapy, with analgesia for the pain.

Following the acute phase and completion of the course of antibiotics, a repeat midstream specimen of urine is obtained and further investigations are carried out to exclude abnormalities of the urinary tract. Acute pyelonephritis may develop into a chronic disease unless the eradication of the infection is complete.

■ Renal failure

Renal failure may be acute or chronic. The former implies the sudden cessation of kidney function and may occur due to a decrease in the blood supply to the kidney. There are many causes of acute renal failure including haemorrhage, plasma loss (burns), acute cardiac failure, dehydration, septicaemia, substances toxic to the kidneys, damage to the kidney substance by disease, interruption to the flow of urine causing obstruction, and crush injuries. The patient with *acute* renal failure goes through two distinct phases, the oliguric phase and the diuretic phase.

□ Oliguric phase

In this phase there is a decreased kidney output and the aims of treatment during this period are to maintain the fluid and electrolyte balance and to keep accumulation of waste products within limits that are compatible with life. This is achieved by rest and restricting the fluids administered to approximately 500ml in 24 hours – this covers the loss of water through the skin and lungs, plus the equivalent of the previous day's output – and restricting protein intake to 20g a day. Adequate calorie intake is maintained by giving fats and carbohydrates to prevent the breakdown of tissue protein; electrolytes are withheld. If nausea and vomiting are a problem the carbohydrates may be administered intravenously. All fluids (oral/ intravenous) and food given to the patient are checked for potassium content. Blood is obtained at frequent regular intervals so that the urea and electrolyte levels are closely monitored, enabling the doctor to estimate the necessary restrictions of fluid and diet. Electrocardiograms (ECG) are performed to monitor any changes in the heart which may occur from potassium intoxication. If the metabolic wastes accumulate and the fluid and electrolyte imbalance are severe, threatening life, peritoneal or haemodialysis may be commenced.

□ Diuretic phase

This is heralded by an increase in the urinary output and signifies that there is some recovery taking place in the kidney tissues. During this phase the patient passes huge volumes of urine as the kidneys are still unable to concentrate, select and conserve electrolytes. Consequently there is loss of excessive amounts of sodium and potassium. The aim of treatment during this phase is to maintain a fluid and electrolyte balance by restoring what has been lost in the urine. The intake of protein in the diet is still regulated and controlled by the urea levels in the blood. Treatment is continued until the kidneys are able to control the volume and composition of urine produced.

☐ *Chronic renal failure*

This is gradual in onset and may be the result of some previous kidney disease, the nephrons progressively becoming permanently damaged. In its early stages the disorder may not be recognizable, as compensation takes place where the work of the damaged nephrons is taken over by others still functioning. When this compensation fails the kidneys are no longer able to maintain a constant internal environment. The aim of treatment is based on the stage of failure and as far as possible the patient's condition is maintained by regulation of the fluid and dietary intake. As the disease progresses to the terminal stages of renal failure, symptoms and signs may include those of the nervous system – muscular twitching, convulsions, drowsiness; the high urea levels irritate the gastro-intestinal tract giving rise to nausea, vomiting, hiccoughs; the patient may have a dry mouth which may become coated with a dirty brown fur; a distortion of the blood pH (acidosis) affects the respiration; the patient becomes anaemic and hypertensive, and there is usually an increase in the volume of urine which contains proteins. The fluid intake is adjusted according to the urinary output, and the dietary protein is usually restricted according to the blood urea levels. Anaemia is usually treated by blood transfusions and hypertension may require drug therapy. When conservative treatment is no longer adequate in maintaining the fluid and electrolyte balance and excretion of waste products, the patient may eventually reach the stage where maintenance of life may only be achieved by regular haemodialysis.

■ RENAL FUNCTION TESTS

These are tests performed to establish the ability of the kidneys to filter and reabsorb substances. They include the estimation of blood urea and blood creatinine levels, urea concentration and urea and creatinine clearance tests, dilution and concentration tests. The specific preparation and management of the patient differs according to the test carried out. In some instances fluids are withheld for a stated number of hours and urine is collected at stated intervals, or all the urine passed during a 24-hour period may be collected. The nurse should be aware of the necessary preparations and be familiar with the laboratory containers necessary. Specimens of blood may also be required to accompany the urine specimens to the laboratory.

■ 24-hour urine collection

This involves the collection of all the urine passed by the patient over a 24-hour period. The collection bottles should be correctly labelled with the patient's name and time of collection. The first specimen of urine obtained at the commencement of the stated time is discarded. All the urine voided for the next 24 hours is collected and the final specimen voided at the end of this period is included in the collection. The need for saving all urine passed is explained to the patient.

■ Midstream specimen of urine (MSU)

This is obtained after cleansing the skin area around the urethral orifice. The patient is asked to void and interrupt the stream so that the middle part is passed into a sterile container. A midstream specimen of urine is required for culture and sensitivity.

Other investigations may include straight abdominal radiographs, intravenous urogram, cystoscopy permitting catheterization of the ureters, retrograde urography, renal angiography and biopsy.

■ DIALYSIS

This may be employed so that the functions of the kidneys can be performed artificially. Dialysis works on the principles of osmosis and diffusion, where two solutions (blood and dialysate) are separated by a semi-permeable membrane and the movement of solutes and fluids is determined by the concentration gradient on either side of the membrane. The semi-permeable membrane may be provided by the patient's own peritoneum, dialysing fluid being passed into the abdominal cavity (peritoneal dialysis), or dialysis may be achieved by the use of a dialysing machine. The patient's blood is passed through a machine containing dialysing fluid and the semi-permeable membrane is provided by special porous cellophane. An atriovenous shunt or an atriovenous fistula is established so that the patient can be attached to a kidney machine.

■ SUMMARY OF NURSING CARE OF PATIENTS WITH DISEASE OF THE KIDNEY

■ Position in the ward

The patient will be placed in a position where he will receive maximum observation. If haemodialysis is required it is carried out in a specialized unit and the patient is under constant observation. Some patients with disease of the kidney, e.g. renal failure, are susceptible to infection and a reverse barrier nursing procedure may be instituted. Safety of the patient should be maintained at all times and should the patient become drowsy or develop convulsions cot sides should be used.

■ Position of patient and mobilization

The patient may be allowed to assume the position in which he is most comfortable. If the patient is very weak and lethargic the nurses should move him at regular intervals to prevent the formation of pressure sores; this is particularly important where the kidneys are failing to function, as breakdown of body tissue increases the levels of potassium in the blood. Appropriate aids may be selected to help prevent the development of pressure sores, e.g. sheepskin. Rest is important to reduce activity, as this affects the production of metabolic wastes. The patient will be allowed to mobilize gradually as his condition responds to treatment. Care should be taken that the patient does not hurt himself when he begins to mobilize. Chest physiotherapy is important and deep breathing and coughing are encouraged to prevent pulmonary complications.

■ Eating and drinking

Many patients suffering from kidney disease may require treatment involving regulation of the diet. The restriction of protein in the diet, leaving mainly carbohydrates and fats, is not very palatable and the nurse must use her skills to make the food appear appetizing and to help the patient with his diet. In acute glomerulonephritis this restriction may be of a relatively short duration, depending on the patient's response to treatment. In other more chronic diseases the diet may have to be tolerated for a longer period of time. The dietician may be asked to talk to the patient about his likes and dislikes in relation to food, and suggest ways in which his diet can be varied within the constraints imposed. Salt may also be restricted from the diet due to sodium retention. Patients with pyelonephritis usually take a light diet while pyrexial and resume their usual diet as their condition improves. The fluid intake for the patient with pyelonephritis is also increased, provided the patient is passing urine. The fluid intake for a patient with renal disease is based on the body's ability to maintain fluid balance and the urinary output. Whether fluids are restricted or given liberally it is important that a strict fluid balance record is kept and that all entries made are accurate. The patient should be observed for any excess perspiration which, if in evidence, should be reported and recorded.

■ Observations

Specific observations of temperature, pulse, respiration and blood pressure should be made at regular and frequent intervals. The temperature is usually raised in acute glomerulonephritis and pyelonephritis. It is also an important observation to make of a patient with a chronic renal disease, as any rise in temperature may signify the onset of an infection. The pulse and respiration rate should be closely observed as changes may occur due to an electrolyte imbalance, cardiac involvement, or a disturbance in the acid-base balance. Hypertension is evident in many renal conditions and is regularly monitored and recorded. It may require antihypertensive therapy.

Continuous observations are made of the patient receiving blood transfusions.

The response of oedema to treatment may be assessed by daily weighing of the patient.

The patient should also be observed for increasing signs of drowsiness and muscular twitching.

■ Skin and general hygiene

If the patient is pyrexial frequent washes should be given to refresh the patient, with changes of bed linen and nightwear. A fan may also be used to keep the patient cool. The condition of the patient's skin must be closely observed as any marks suggestive of pressure may indicate the need for more frequent moving and lifting of the patient. If the patient is perspiring freely more frequent washes should be given. A high blood urea level may give rise to pruritus and the application of calamine lotion may give some relief for the patient. The skin may become dry and, as it may excrete substances normally excreted by the kidneys, may become a yellowish/brownish colour. If urea is present in the sweat it occasionally crystallizes on the skin giving the appearance of what is termed 'urea frost'.

Care of the patient's mouth is necessary and measures are taken to keep the mouth clean and moist when, as in acute glomerulonephritis, fluids are withheld and the patient is pyrexial. Frequent brushing of teeth and mouthwashes should be given and a substance applied to the lips to prevent drying and cracking. When the kidneys are failing the greatest care must be taken of the patient's mouth as the salivary secretion is reduced, crusts may develop on the dry mucosa and lips, the tongue may become coated and ulcers may develop. If the urea level is considerably raised the patient may complain of an 'offensive' taste in his mouth. Boiled sweets may be useful in stimulating salivary gland secretions and in keeping the mouth moist.

■ **Elimination**

All urine passed should be measured and accurately recorded. Urine may have to be tested daily for the presence of protein and specimens obtained at intervals for laboratory investigation. The nurse should be familiar with laboratory instructions governing the collection of specific specimens. The appearance of the urine should be noted and frequently it is necessary to obtain the specific gravity. A record of the urinary output is necessary for the doctor to estimate the regulation of fluid intake. Efforts are made to prevent the development of constipation and any diarrhoea present is recorded and reported.

■ **Administration of drugs**

They will be administered as prescribed by the doctor and will vary considerably between renal diseases. Generally the drugs which may be prescribed for acute glomerulonephritis and pyelonephritis are antibiotics, and possibly analgesia for any pain which may accompany pyelonephritis. The drugs prescribed for the chronic renal diseases are dependent on the condition of the patient, the stage of the disease and the degree of renal insufficiency. They may include antihypertensive drugs, and, as high blood urea levels irritate the mucosa of the gastro-intestinal tracts, antacids may be given orally. Analgesia may be prescribed if pain is present, e.g. in acute renal failure following trauma or surgery. The patient may also complain of headaches. Drugs may also be required to alleviate nausea, vomiting and persistent hiccoughs, e.g. chlorpromazine. An ion exchange resin may also be prescribed to prevent the absorption of potassium from the gastro-intestinal tract; it may be administered orally or rectally.

For complications which may arise following acute renal failure, involving the heart, lungs or possibly convulsions, the doctor will prescribe the appropriate drugs.

When patients have a disease affecting renal function, particularly renal insufficiency, regular and frequent assessment of the blood urea, electrolyte levels, pH and urinary output is of paramount importance. The results of the findings should be placed where they are easily available to the medical and nursing staff for frequent reference.

■ **Advice to patient and relatives**

The more the patient and the relatives understand about renal disease the better, as much co-operation is required by them in terms of adapting their activity, diets and occupation. The importance of regular, frequent check-ups is emphasized and the patient with chronic renal failure, for example, will be required to observe his urinary output and, if any significant changes occur, he is advised to see the doctor. Whether the patient can continue with his occupation will depend on his condition and the demands of the job, and as the chronic diseases may require periodic admissions into hospital the family may encounter financial difficulties. The medical social worker may be asked to discuss the situation with them if they so desire.

■ PRACTICE QUESTIONS

1 *What is meant by the following terms?*
   a Nephron.
   b Glomerular filtration.
   c Tubular reabsorption.
   d Tubular secretion.
   e Antidiuretic hormone.
   f Aldosterone.
   g Erythropoietin.
   h Renin.
   i Polyuria.
   j Micturition.
   k Acute glomerulonephritis.
   l Uraemia.
   m Renal failure.
   n Oliguria.
   o Haemodialysis.
2 *Briefly explain the following:*
   a Why anaemia is associated with chronic renal disease.
   b Why it is necessary during the diuretic phase of acute renal failure to regulate the fluid intake and monitor electrolyte balance when the patient is producing a diuresis.
   c Why a restricted protein diet is instituted for the treatment of acute glomerulonephritis.
   d How a patient would be prepared for an intravenous urogram.
   e The importance of recording accurate fluid balance when a patient has renal insufficiency.
3 *Determine whether or not the following statements are true or false:*
   a The glomerular filtration rate is the rate at which the urine flows through the renal tubules.
   b Each nephron produces 1ml of urine per minute.

c Tubular reabsorption allows for substances needed by the body to be taken back from the tubules.

d The efferent arteriole carries blood to the glomerulus of the nephron.

e Haemodialysis can be employed to remove excess fluid which has accumulated in the body, as well as electrolytes and nitrogenous waste products of metabolism.

f Because hydrogen ions are not eliminated by the renal tubules when a patient is in renal failure he may develop metabolic acidosis.

g Crush injuries may cause acute renal failure and are associated with the increase of myohaemoglobin in the circulation.

■ **Answers**

1 a The functioning unit of the kidney necessary for the formation of urine.

b The process of filtering the blood which takes place in the glomerulus.

c Certain substances filtered by the glomerulus are reabsorbed by the capillary network surrounding the renal tubules. The substances reabsorbed are selected according to the needs of the body.

d The ability of the tubular cells to secrete substances into the glomerular filtrate. The substances are actively transported by the cells of the tubule.

e Antidiuretic hormone (ADH) from the posterior pituitary gland. Its release is controlled by the hypothalamus and it regulates the reabsorption of water in the renal tubules.

f Aldosterone is a hormone produced by the adrenal cortex which increases the reabsorption of sodium by the renal tubules.

g A hormone-like substance produced by the kidneys, necessary for the formation of red blood cells.

h A protein splitting enzyme released into the blood by the kidneys in response to an inadequate blood flow to the kidneys.

i A significant and persistent increase in the volume of urinary output.

j The process of voiding urine.

k Inflammation of the glomerulus of the kidneys. It frequently follows an upper respiratory tract infection with *Haemolytic streptococcus*.

l Refers to an increase in the amount of urea retained in the blood, and excessive substances which are usually excreted by the kidneys.

m The kidneys are failing to function and are therefore unable to maintain a suitable environment for the body cells.

n A decrease in the urinary output which may be due to kidney disease, or a decreased blood flow to the kidney, e.g. congestive cardiac failure or hypotension.

o The accumulated waste products of metabolism and electrolytes are removed from the body by the artificial kidney machine. This involves extending the patient's circulation by means of tubing and the passage of blood (in the tube) through a machine containing dialysing fluid. The patient's blood is separated from the fluid by a semi-permeable membrane.

2 a The origin of the anaemia is uncertain but it is thought that it may be due to a deficiency of erythropoetin. The anaemia is usually treated by a slow transfusion of blood as the anaemia does not usually respond to iron therapy.

b This is because, although urinary output is increased, the kidneys have not recovered sufficiently to be selective in terms of what is retained by the body and what is excreted, so that laboratory analysis of the blood levels of urea and electrolytes have to be continued, and the fluid and dietary intake regulated accordingly.

c The glomeruli of the kidneys are inflamed and they are responsible for excreting the waste products of protein metabolism (urea creatinine, uric acid). Restricting the intake of protein ensures some rest for the kidneys to aid recovery, and prevents the accumulation of these products in the body from where the kidneys may be unable to excrete them in sufficient quantities.

d The nature of the procedure is explained to the patient. Check that the patient has no allergies. Fluids are withheld for approximately 12 hours, but a dry breakfast may be given if the patient so desires. Suppositories may be given the night prior to the investigation as the presence of gas and faeces may interfere with the radiological examination. A gown is placed on the patient, secured by ties.

e The kidneys normally maintain the internal environment of the body cells by regulating the fluid balance. This regulating mechanism is lost if the kidneys are not functioning adequately. Fluid balance therefore has to be maintained; the doctor relies on the nurses to measure all fluid intake and output so that he or she can prescribe the administration of the appropriate type and amount of fluids to maintain a fluid balance compatible with life.

3 a False
b False
c True
d False
e True
f True
g True

6 The liver and hepatitis

The purpose of this chapter is to indicate:
1 The structure and functions of the liver.
2 The types of jaundice.
3 The total management of a patient with hepatitis.

■ THE LIVER

The liver is a large reddish brown wedge-shaped organ situated on the right-hand side in the upper abdomen, beneath the diaphragm. It is covered by peritoneum, except for a bare area on the posterior surface which is closely related to the diaphragm.

The blood supply providing oxygen for the liver cells is by way of the hepatic artery. Blood is also brought to the liver by the portal vein which carries blood rich in food materials absorbed by the gut, and insulin from the pancreas. Blood leaves the liver via the hepatic veins which drain into the inferior vena cava.

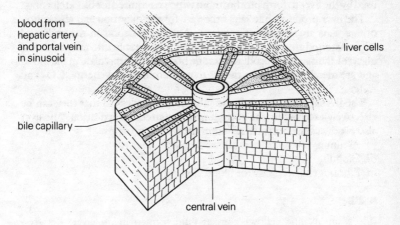

blood from hepatic artery and portal vein in sinusoid

liver cells

bile capillary

central vein

Fig. 5 Liver lobule illustrating arrangement of cells around a central vein

Microscopically the liver can be seen to be arranged into lobules (Fig. 5). The liver cells are arranged in chains and each chain has a blood sinusoid on one side and a bile capillary on the other. These structures are arranged in a circle around a central vein.

As the blood passes through the sinusoids (from the hepatic artery and portal vein) it is in direct contact with the liver cells. The portal vein provides the liver cells with absorbed substances which undergo further changes in the liver, and the hepatic artery supplies the liver cells with the oxygen necessary for this cellular activity. The liver has many functions and is essential for life.

■ Changes in foodstuffs in the liver

□ *Proteins*
The de-amination of surplus amino acids produces ammonia and this is converted by the liver cells into urea, which is then excreted by the kidneys.

□ *Carbohydrates*
Glucose is stored as glycogen in the liver, and is used to maintain the blood glucose levels. The hormones adrenaline and glucagon convert liver glycogen into blood glucose.

□ *Fats*
The fat soluble vitamins A, D, E and K are stored in the liver. Vitamin K is used by the liver to form prothrombin which is required for blood clotting.

The liver produces bile salts necessary for the digestion and absorption of fats. Fats are stored in the liver and other fat depots in the body and when required are taken to the liver where they are split into fatty acids and glycerol. This process produces ketone bodies which circulate in the blood and are metabolized by the tissues to produce heat and energy, CO_2 and water.

The liver renders certain toxic substances harmless so that they can be effectively excreted by the body, a process termed detoxication. The liver also produces bile and manufactures the plasma proteins:
  i Albumin
 ii Globulin
iii Fibrinogen (necessary for blood clotting).

■ Bile

Bile is an alkaline yellowish-green fluid formed in the liver. Between 500–1000ml of bile is secreted daily, containing water, calcium and sodium salts, and bile pigments. The bile salts are formed from sodium salts combining with certain amino acids in the liver. They activate pancreatic lipase and are necessary for the digestion and absorption of fats. Bile salts are recycled during the process of digestion and are taken back to the liver from the small intestine via the portal vein for re-secretion. The small amounts of bile salts lost in the faeces are replaced by the liver cells.

Bile pigments bilirubin and biliverdin are formed from broken-down red blood cells. At the end of their 120-days life span the red blood cells are taken up by the cells of the reticulo-endothelial system. Part of the cell is broken down into amino acids and iron and stored in the body, the remainder is converted into bile pigments. The bile pigments are transported to the liver by the blood combined with plasma albumin because at this stage the bilirubin is not soluble in water. As the bilirubin passes through the liver cells the albumin is removed and replaced by an acid formed from glucose; this renders the pigments water soluble and they are then transferred to the bile ducts as post-hepatic bilirubin. The bilirubin is excreted in bile via the hepatic ducts and common bile duct to the duodenum and large intestine, where the bilirubin is converted to stercobilinogen under the influence of bacterial action, giving faeces their characteristic brown colour. Some of the bilirubin is reabsorbed as it passes through the large intestine and is excreted in the urine as urobilinogen. Bile is stored and concentrated in the gall bladder and when food, particularly fats, enters the duodenum the mucosa releases the hormone cholecystokinin stimulating the release of bile from the gall bladder.

■ JAUNDICE (Fig. 6)

This is the term given to the yellow discolouration of the skin which develops when there is an increased accumulation of bile pigments and salts in the blood. If the pathway for the excretion of bilirubin fails or is obstructed, jaundice may develop. There may be excessive breakdown of red blood cells which will give rise to *haemolytic jaundice*. Derangement of the liver cells due to damage to, or disease of, the liver tissue will give rise to *hepatic jaundice*. Obstruction to the flow of bile from the liver to the intestine will cause *obstructive jaundice*.

■ Haemolytic jaundice

Due to the excessive destruction of red blood cells there is an accumulation of bilirubin in the blood giving rise to jaundice. This is not usually severe as the liver can cope with the increase. However, the increased amounts are excreted via the hepatic ducts to the intestines and an increased amount of stercobilinogen is produced, giving rise to dark faeces. Excessive amounts

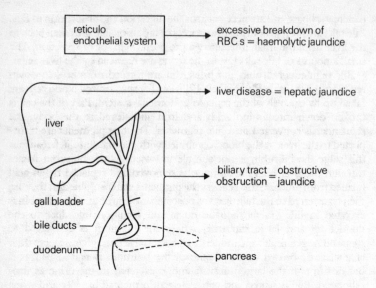

Fig. 6 The types of jaundice

of urobilinogen are also formed and excreted in the urine. As bile salts are being excreted normally there is usually no pruritus.

■ Obstructive jaundice

Due to the obstruction to the flow of bile, the water-soluble bilirubin and other substances found in bile are reabsorbed into the bloodstream, giving rise to a jaundice which may be very deep. The excessive bilirubin in the blood is excreted in the urine, giving rise to dark coloured urine. Due to the obstruction bilirubin does not get through to the intestine. This causes a deficiency in stercobilinogen, resulting in the passage of pale clay-coloured stools which contain large amounts of fat. The accumulation of bile salts in the blood causes pruritus and sometimes the patient is found to have a decreased pulse rate. Deficiency of vitamin K (fat soluble vitamin) occurs, as it requires bile salts for its absorption. This deficiency gives rise to a tendency to haemorrhage.

■ Hepatic jaundice

This develops following damage to the liver cells by toxic substances or infection. The liver cells are unable to transfer the bilirubin from the blood to the bile ducts. The degree of jaundice depends on the damage to the liver; if the liver cells become very swollen and inflamed the patient manifests all the symptoms of obstructive jaundice.

ACUTE HEPATITIS

This is the term used for inflammation of the liver, most commonly caused by viruses. The virus which causes *acute infective hepatitis* is the A virus; that which causes *serum hepatitis* is the B virus. The two differ mainly in the way they are transmitted and the incubation period.

The A virus causing infective hepatitis is present in faeces and is transmitted in contaminated water or food. It may also be present in the blood and urine and may therefore be transmitted by contaminated syringes or needles, or through infected blood or plasma. The incubation period is between 15 and 50 days.

The B virus causing serum hepatitis appears to be more virulent than the A virus and is transmitted by infected blood plasma or serum, or by contaminated syringes or needles. It has been found that a large proportion of patients with serum hepatitis have the Australia antigen present in their blood, and blood taken from donors who are Australia antigen positive has resulted in a high incidence of serum hepatitis. Outbreaks of hepatitis in haemodialysis units have also led to the detection of the Australia antigen. Serum hepatitis usually has a longer incubation period but may range from 15–100 days.

The signs and symptoms caused by virus A and virus B are similar but the incidence of infective hepatitis is higher among children and young adults. The patient usually complains of feeling generally unwell, with headaches, nausea, vomiting, loss of appetite and vague abdominal pains; constipation or diarrhoea may develop, and pyrexia may be present. Some patients may present with severe abdominal pain. Tenderness is observed in the region of the liver and jaundice may be detected, with the presence of bile in the urine. If an obstruction to the flow of bile develops in the liver the jaundice becomes deeper, the stools lighter, the urine darker, and the liver enlarges. In the majority of patients the signs and symptoms subside and the patient makes a complete recovery. Occasionally a patient may go on to develop chronic hepatic insufficiency.

There is no specific treatment for acute hepatitis and care is largely supportive. The investigations include liver function tests and abdominal radiological examination, urinalysis, and examination of blood for Australia antigen.

■ SUMMARY OF NURSING CARE OF PATIENTS WITH DISEASE OF THE LIVER

■ Position of patient on the ward

The patient with viral hepatitis is placed in a single-bedded side room and barrier nursing procedures are instituted. The correct use of gowns and gloves, cleansing of hands, and the disposal of linen and excreta are of great importance. Care should be taken with the collection of blood specimens and their transportation to the laboratory; the local policy should be adhered to in relation to this, as well as correct disposal of the syringes, needles and intravenous giving sets.

■ Eating and drinking

If the patient can tolerate food a high calorie diet may be recommended. However, the patient may be better able to tolerate a light diet supplemented with fruit drinks and glucose. Depending on the patient's ability to tolerate food, nutrients may have to be administered by intravenous infusion. Fats are not usually tolerated until the condition improves. An increased fluid intake is necessary as the patient may be pyrexial, and also to promote elimination of bilirubin in the urine. Disposable crockery and utensils should be used.

■ Skin and general hygiene

Frequent washes to keep the patient cool and refreshed are required while the patient is pyrexial, with adequate changes of linen. Soap should be used sparingly as it may aggravate the pruritus which may be present. The application of calamine lotion may have a soothing effect on the skin. Nails should be kept clean and short to avoid skin abrasions through scratching. The mouth should be kept clean and moist, and if the patient is well enough to clean his own teeth he should be provided with the appropriate facilities. Care should be taken with nasal and mouth secretions and used tissues should be correctly disposed of.

■ Position in bed and mobilization

The patient will assume the position in which he is most comfortable. A back rest and pillows can be used during the day to support the patient in a sitting position and, if he prefers, these can be removed for sleeping during the night. Rest in bed is usually maintained for approximately 2–3 weeks until the patient's appetite is improved, and the liver is no longer enlarged and the jaundice subsided. If the patient is very weak he should be moved by nurses and have his position changed frequently; if the patient is strong enough the importance of changing position in bed is explained and he is encouraged to move himself. The skin is closely observed for redness at regular intervals, and more frequent changes of position are employed if required. The mobilization of the patient is gradual, at first sitting the patient in a chair for short periods, gradually increasing the time; the walking distance is gradually increased according to the patient's condition. Deep breathing and leg exercises are encouraged and supervised while the patient remains on bed rest.

■ Elimination

All faeces must be disposed of correctly, adhering to the hospital procedure. Depending on the facilities available for the disposal of excreta, the faeces may require treatment with disinfectant prior to their disposal. The greatest care must be taken in preventing contamination with excreta; the nurse should protect herself by wearing gloves for all procedures which involve possible contamination, e.g. the administration of an enema. Care should also be taken in the handling and disposal of urine and gloves should be worn for the purpose of urinalysis.

■ Observations

The temperature should be taken and recorded at regular intervals according to the patient's condition. The patient should have his own thermometer which should preferably be discarded on his discharge from hospital, due to the difficulty of sterilizing thermometers. Alternatively, disposable thermometers may be used. The pulse rate and blood pressure are observed at appropriate intervals. The skin is observed for signs of pruritus and the degree of jaundice present is noted.

A record of the fluid balance is continued during the acute stage and also while the patient is receiving intravenous therapy. The patient will be weighed daily if the doctor suspects that fluid is being retained.

Note should be made of the patient's appetite as it is important to maintain a good nutritional state to ensure recovery. If the patient is found not to be taking his diet, the reasons for this should be obtained and, if necessary, the dietician may be asked to discuss with the patient his likes and dislikes.

The patient's mood should be observed because complete recovery may take some time and, as a result, the patient may feel persistently tired and somewhat depressed. Measures should be taken to ascertain what the patient's interests are; as he regains his strength, and during the convalescent period, he may continue with these interests to prevent boredom.

As the patient may have a tendency to bleed during the course of illness, observation should be made of these signs and any abnormalities reported.

■ **Administration of drugs**

There is no specific drug used in the treatment of hepatitis and care is taken when drugs are prescribed because of the important function of the liver in the modification and detoxication of many drugs. Due to disease the duration of action of some drugs may be unduly prolonged. Occasionally prednisone may be prescribed if, after a number of weeks, the patient remains deeply jaundiced.

■ **Communication**

The patient is kept informed of progress and the necessity for barrier nursing is explained to both the patient and his relatives. The necessity for the highest standard of hygiene is explained and the patient's co-operation is sought.

The need for a long period of convalescence is discussed with the patient and his family and they are advised that, should the patient's symptoms recur, he should consult the doctor and a further period of bed rest may be required. During discussions the family should realize that the period of convalescence may not be without some difficulty, as the patient may become irritable when he feels he is capable of doing more than he is allowed. The patient is advised to refrain from taking alcohol for approximately 3–6 months.

■ TESTS WHICH MAY BE CARRIED OUT TO AID DIAGNOSIS IN LIVER DISEASE

Liver function tests are carried out to monitor the progress of liver disease as well as to determine the presence and degree of any disorder. They include specific tests performed on blood and urine. The amounts of bilirubin can be measured in the blood, faeces and urine. The quantitative van den Bergh test measures the amount of serum bilirubin and can differentiate between bilirubin soluble in water and that which is insoluble. The latter is bound to protein and it is necessary to remove the protein to determine the amount of bilirubin. This is known as the *indirect* van den Bergh reaction. The amount of water-soluble bilirubin is determined by the *direct* van den Bergh reaction. Prothrombin levels may be determined when liver disease is suspected as it is normally manufactured by the liver. Tests may also be performed to assess the liver's ability to metabolize proteins, and to maintain the normal levels of plasma proteins.

Ammonia levels, when raised, are indicative of hepatic insufficiency as the liver normally converts ammonia into urea.

Tests may also be carried out to determine the level of carbohydrate and lipid metabolism.

It is also possible to test the liver's ability to detoxify and excrete substances. Other tests involve estimation of the serum enzyme levels, serum cholinesterase and alkaline phosphatase tests.

Abdominal radiological examination and special radio-isotope scanning techniques may also be employed, and biopsy of the liver may be performed.

■ PRACTICE QUESTIONS

1 *What is meant by the following terms?*
   a Right hypochondrium.
   b Bile.
   c Detoxication.
   d Glycogen.
   e Haemolytic jaundice.
   f Obstructive jaundice.
   g Viral hepatitis.
   h Liver failure.
   i Stercobilinogen.
   j Fat soluble vitamins.
   k Bile salts.
   l Prothrombin.
   m Ketone bodies.
   n Ammonia.
   o Glucagon.
   p Ascites.

2 *Briefly explain the following:*
   a How bile is released from the gall bladder to pass down the common bile duct into the duodenum.
   b The most common causes of obstructive jaundice.
   c Why there is an excessive amount of urobilinogen present in the urine of a patient with haemolytic jaundice.
   d Why a patient with obstructive jaundice may have a prolonged clotting time.

  e Why pruritus may be a problem in obstructive jaundice and not in haemolytic jaundice.

  f Why people who are Australia antigen positive should not become blood donors.

  g Why ascites may develop in a person with a chronic hepatic disease such as cirrhosis of the liver.

3 Describe the total management of a patient undergoing paracentesis abdominis.

4 *Mark the following statements true or false:*

  a Cells of the reticulo-endothelial system which destroy red blood cells are found in the liver as well as the spleen and bone marrow.

  b Primary carcinoma of the liver is common.

  c It is believed that the accumulation of bile salts in the blood causes bradycardia.

  d Adrenaline causes conversion of liver glycogen into glucose.

  e A patient in liver failure would have a high blood urea level.

  f The Australia antigen is associated with virus A causing hepatitis.

  g Bile salts and pancreatic lipase are necessary for the digestion and absorption of fats.

  h Apparently healthy persons may be carriers of the type A and B viruses of hepatitis.

■ **Answers**

1 *a* A specific division of the abdomen. The abdominal divisions are used to locate certain abdominal organs.

  b A yellowish-green alkaline fluid formed in the liver.

  c By changing the chemical composition of some substances they can be made less harmful.

  d Glucose converted so that it can be stored in the body either as liver glycogen or muscle glycogen.

  e Jaundice due to excessive breakdown of red blood cells with subsequent excessive levels of bile pigments.

  f Jaundice which develops due to the obstruction to the flow of bile from the liver to the duodenum.

  g Inflammation of the liver caused by a virus.

  h Due to disease of, or damage to, the liver cells the organ is unable to carry out its normal functions.

  i The action of bacteria on bilirubin in the large intestine converts it to stercobilinogen which gives faeces their normal brown colour.

  j Insoluble in water and require bile salts for their absorption.

  k Formed in the liver and contained in bile. They are necessary for the digestion and absorption of fats.

l A plasma protein formed in the liver from vitamin K and required for blood clotting.

m Formed by the liver as a result of fat metabolism.

n Ammonia is formed as a result of protein metabolism.

o Hormone produced by the alpha cells of the islets of Langerhans which is required for the conversion of liver glycogen to glucose.

p Formation of fluid in the peritoneal cavity.

2 *a* The gall bladder contracts in response to the hormone cholecystokinin.

b Obstruction or disease of the liver,
e.g. inflammation
cirrhosis
carcinoma
Obstruction in the biliary tract,
e.g. gallstones
strictures
Pressure from outside on the biliary tract,
e.g. carcinoma of head of pancreas.

c Although excess bilirubin is formed, there is no obstruction to the flow of bile and the excess therefore passes through to the intestines. The excess stercobilinogen formed increases the amount of urobilinogen absorbed and excreted in the urine.

d Due to obstruction bile salts are not getting through to the duodenum and vitamin K is not absorbed. The liver requires vitamin K (fat soluble vitamin) for the production of prothrombin.

e It is believed that pruritus is caused by the accumulation of bile salts and if there is an obstruction present they, as well as bilirubin, will accumulate in the blood. Although in haemolytic jaundice there are excess bile pigments being produced, bile salts do not accumulate as there is no obstruction preventing them from passing through to the duodenum as they would normally.

f The Australia antigen is associated with serum hepatitis.

g Inability of the liver to produce adequate albumin, thereby disturbing the plasma osmotic pressure. Increased pressure in the portal vein. Ascites disturbs the fluid balance in the body bringing into play compensatory mechanisms such as antidiuretic hormone and aldosterone production which increases the ascites.

3 The following points should be considered when a patient is undergoing a paracentesis abdominis:
Explanation of procedure to the patient. Position patient. Sitting position with the back supported by pillows. The patient's arms should lie on either side.

Empty bladder prior to procedure.

Preparation of equipment to include local anaesthetic for insertion of trocar and cannula and adequate tubing and bags for the fluid withdrawn.

Preparation of abdomen – shaving and cleansing.

Patient should be closely observed throughout the procedure for colour, pulse and blood pressure; a sphygmomanometer cuff may be applied to the arm before the procedure begins.

Removal of too much fluid too quickly may lead to circulatory failure and shock and it is usual, therefore, not to remove more than 1 to 2 litres at a time.

Plasma or whole blood transfusion may be necessary following the procedure to replace the proteins lost in the fluid withdrawn.

The fluid obtained is inspected and measured.

On completion of the procedure a sterile dressing is placed over the puncture site and an abdominal binder applied.

The patient assumes the supine position and observations of pulse and blood pressure are continued at frequent intervals for a number of hours.

The equipment is correctly disposed of.

It may be necessary for one nurse to remain with the patient throughout the procedure while a second nurse assists the doctor.

4 *a* True
   b False
   c True
   d True
   e False
   f False
   g True
   h True

7 Thyrotoxicosis/diabetes mellitus

The purpose of this chapter is to indicate:
1 The structure and function of the thyroid gland and the islets of Langerhans.
2 The management of patients with thyrotoxicosis or diabetes mellitus.

■ THE THYROID GLAND

The thyroid gland is a V-shaped organ situated in the lower neck in front of the trachea. It consists of two lobes which are joined together in the centre by the isthmus. The lobes consist of many follicles lined with secreting thyroid cells which are cuboid in shape. Contained in the follicles is a clear viscous colloidal substance called thyroglobulin. (Other endocrine glands store their hormones in the cells.) The gland receives a good blood supply via the inferior and superior thyroid arteries which are branches of the subclavian and external carotid arteries respectively. The four parathyroid glands are situated posteriorly to the thyroid gland and they also receive their blood supply from the two pairs of thyroid arteries. The recurrent laryngeal nerves are closely related to the gland posteriorly.

The thyroid gland requires iodine in order to produce the hormone thyroxine which is in two related forms, according to the number of iodine atoms that it contains, thyroxine (T_4) or tri-iodothyronine (T_3). The release to thyroxine is under the control of the thyroid stimulating hormone (TSH) from the anterior pituitary gland. The TSH in turn is under the influence of the thyroid stimulating hormone releasing factor from the hypothalamus (TSH-RF). The action of TSH and TSH-RF is dependent on the levels of circulating thyroxine. A constant level of thyroxine can therefore be maintained by this feedback mechanism.

> →Hypothalamus – Releasing factor (TSH-RF)
> ↓
> →Anterior Pituitary – Thyroid stimulating hormone (TSH)
> ↓
> →Thyroid Gland – Thyroxine (T_4) Tri-iodothyronine (T_3)

The thyroid gland also produces a hormone called calcitonin which lowers the blood calcium levels.

Enlargement of the thyroid gland (goitre) may be due to iodine deficiency.

Underactivity of the thyroid gland gives rise to the condition myxoedema in adults when the blood level of thyroxine falls.

Overactivity of the thyroid gland causes hyperthyroidism; when a person becomes ill due to the increase in the metabolic rate, thyrotoxicosis describes the condition. The function of thyroxine is to increase the metabolic rate of all the body cells.

■ THYROTOXICOSIS

Thyrotoxicosis is also known as toxic goitre, exophthalmic goitre and Graves' disease. Due to the increase in the amount of thyroxine produced and a general increase in metabolic activity, the skin becomes hot and sweaty as more heat is produced. The patient may lose weight as food is rapidly converted to heat, even though the appetite remains good. The heart rate is increased and the sleeping pulse raised, and atrial fibrillation may develop. Palpitations may also be present. The patient may be unduly nervous, apprehensive and restless, and a fine tremor of the hands may be observed when the arms are outstretched. Increased activity of the gastro-intestinal tract may give rise to diarrhoea, and amenorrhoea may be a feature in female patients. The thyroid gland may be enlarged and exophthalmos (protrusion of the eyeballs) may be present. The patient may also suffer from 'lid-lag' which is a term used for failure of the eyelids to follow the movement of the eyes when the patient looks down. The exophthalmos may be due to a substance (not yet identified) produced by the anterior pituitary and known as the exophthalmic substance.

The disease is commoner in young adult females than in males. There may be a genetic factor associated with thyrotoxicosis, but the exact cause is unknown.

■ Specific investigations

Specific investigations may be carried out to assess the activity of the thyroid gland. The basal metabolic rate (BMR) may be a guide to the activity of the gland. The blood cholesterol levels are usually lowered in thyrotoxicosis.

The serum protein-bound iodine test (PBI) may be carried out to establish the amount of thyroxine in the circulation, since it is bound to plasma protein. The results may be misleading if the patient has received iodine in the form of medication or prior to special radiological procedures involving the use of radio-opaque contrast dyes. The PBI is high in patients with thyrotoxicosis.

Radio-active iodine metabolism is assessed by the use of radio-active isotopes and iodine (I^{132}) and (I^{131}). The radio-activity can be measured directly by the use of a geiger counter over the neck, and indirect measurement may be obtained by estimating the amount of radio-active iodine excreted in the urine in 24 or 48 hours.

The tendon achilles reflex is more rapid with a greater response in patients who are thyrotoxic.

■ Treatment

a Surgical (see the *Surgical Nursing* book in this series).
b Antithyroid drugs.
c Radioactive iodine (I^{131}).

Antithyroid drugs interfere with the formation of the thyroid hormone. Carbimazole is an example of an antithyroid drug which is frequently used. An explanation should be given to the patient regarding the importance of taking the drug at the intervals prescribed. The patient usually begins with a fairly large dose for about 6–8 weeks until an improvement is noted, and then a regular maintenance dose is prescribed. The patient may experience a relapse and a further course of treatment may be necessary, or possibly surgical treatment will be advised and this will be discussed with the patient.

Other alternative drugs that may be prescribed include propylthiouracil and potassium perchlorate. Enlargement of the gland may occur as a result of treatment with antithyroid drugs. This is not considered harmful as long as it does not cause respiratory embarrassment.

Side-effects which may develop as a result of antithyroid drugs include agranulocytosis, hepatitis, dermatitis, diarrhoea, nausea and vomiting.

Phenobarbitone may also be prescribed, with the appropriate antithyroid drug.

If surgical treatment is unsuitable and permanent use of antithyroid drugs is not practical, treatment may be given using radio-active iodine (I^{131}). After oral administration this accumulates in the thyroid gland and destroys the hyperactive tissue.

■ Thyrotoxic crisis

Thyrotoxic crisis is a rare but dangerous complication of uncontrolled hyperthyroidism. It may occur as a result of thyroid surgery, emotional stress, or intercurrent infection. It is thought to be due to the sudden release of increased amounts of thyroxine into the circulation, causing a sudden rapid rise in the metabolic rate. It is manifested by a tachycardia, hyperpyrexia, diarrhoea, nausea, vomiting, apprehension, restlessness and disorientation. The patient may become comatosed and die from heart failure.

Treatment depends on the manifestations but may include intravenous fluids, antithyroid drugs, oxygen, cardiac drugs, sedatives, hydrocortisone. Measures may be taken to cool the patient down and lower his temperature, using ice packs, or by tepid sponging and the use of an electric fan.

■ SUMMARY OF NURSING CARE OF THE PATIENT WITH THYROTOXICOSIS

■ Position on the ward

This is a very important consideration for a patient with thyrotoxicosis. Due to the marked apprehension, irritability and restlessness he should be allowed to remain in a quiet, calm atmosphere which may best be provided in a single side room. If this is not possible great consideration must be given to the placement of the patient in the general ward. Until treatment is established the patient may find it difficult to cope if he is next to a very talkative or very ill patient. The patient should be prepared for tests or investigations in a calm manner, and adequate time should be allowed for this to avoid unnecessary rushing which might increase the patient's apprehension.

■ Position in bed and mobilization

It may not be necessary for the patient to remain on complete bed rest, indeed he may feel better able to relax if allowed to get up and walk about the room, taking rest by sitting in a comfortable chair. The patient should be encouraged to continue with his or her interests, such as reading, listening to the radio, knitting or any other suitable activity. Aimless walking around should be avoided as it will cause the patient to use up a lot of energy. If continued bed rest is necessary the patient's co-operation is sought in regularly changing his position, and comfort is maintained by the use of adequate pillows and a backrest. The patient may also feel more comfortable if he has two or three pillows on which to sleep, rather than lying flat.

■ Eating and drinking

The diet should be discussed with the patient and his likes and dislikes should be established and noted. The nurse should ensure that the patient is not given foods that he has made clear he does not like. The diet should be high in calories, proteins and carbohydrates because of the increased metabolic needs. To meet the patient's appetite a snack may be given at bedtime as the last meal may have been given early in the evening.

Fluid intake is increased to compensate for the fluid lost in perspiration and to enhance the elimination of metabolic wastes by the kidneys.

Decaffeinated coffee may also be made available for the patient.

■ Observations

These include observation at regular intervals of temperature, pulse and respiration. The sleeping pulse rate may also be observed. However, due to the effects of thyroxine, the patient may be a light sleeper and it may therefore prove difficult to obtain the sleeping pulse rate. Anything which causes or increases the patient's restlessness and agitation should be noted and avoided. A check may also be kept on the patient's weight by weighing him daily, or on alternate days. An electrocardiogram may be performed on admission. The reasons for continued observations should always be explained to the patient as lack of understanding may increase his anxiety.

■ Elimination

If the patient is on bed rest he may be allowed up to go to the toilet. If the patient is upset by frequent bowel movements consideration should be given to the proximity of the bathroom and toilet to the patient's bed.

Urinalysis should be performed as glycosuria is sometimes found to be present. Urine may have to be collected for 24-hour urine specimens, and the need to save the urine must be explained to the patient.

■ Administration of drugs

Drugs are administered as prescribed by the doctor. Drugs may also be prescribed to ensure a good night's sleep. Eyedrops may be required to treat the 'grittiness' of the eyes experienced by patients with exophthalmos. When the patient is discharged home on antithyroid drugs he should be told that if he experiences a sore throat, skin rash, swollen nodes (glands) or generally does not feel well he must report the matter to the doctor immediately.

■ **Skin and general hygiene**

The amount of help the patient requires in maintaining his own personal hygiene has to be carefully assessed. The patient should be allowed to wash and care for himself as far as he is able, and at a time when he is least likely to be disturbed in the bathroom. The patient may at times feel embarrassed by his own clumsiness due to tremor, and the nurse should then help the patient in an unobtrusive manner, perhaps by helping with buttoning of clothing while conversing with the patient. If the patient is confined to bed a bed bath may be given daily because of excessive perspiration. The skin should be checked frequently and bedclothes kept loose and to a minimum.

■ **Communication**

The patient should be kept fully informed at all times about his treatment and it should be explained why rest is so important. Involvement of the relatives is important, and they should also understand the need for calm and for avoiding unnecessarily upsetting or arguing with the patient. The relatives should also understand that irritability and agitation shown by the patient are characteristic of the illness, and by being aware of the patient's needs they will be able to help considerably at home. If the patient is found to be agitated as a result of receiving visitors, such visits may have to be limited.

■ DIABETES MELLITUS

This condition develops as a result of the pancreas not producing sufficient insulin to allow glucose to enter the body cells.

■ **The pancreas**

The pancreas is a large gland situated in the abdominal cavity which has both endocrine and exocrine functions. The exocrine functions are performed by the acini cells which secrete pancreatic juice containing enzymes for the process of digestion in the small intestine. Scattered among these cells are groups of smaller cells whose function is endocrine. These are termed the islets of Langerhans. Two types of cells are found in the islets, the alpha and beta cells. The former produce the hormone glucagon, the latter the hormone insulin.

Blood supply to the pancreas is from the coeliac artery via branches of the hepatic and splenic arteries.

■ Insulin

Diabetes mellitus affects the metabolism of carbohydrates and the inability to metabolize carbohydrates effectively subsequently affects the metabolism of fats and proteins.

The presence of insulin is necessary to convert the blood glucose into liver and muscle glycogen. The release of insulin is regulated by the levels of glucose in the blood; for the brain to function normally a level of 3.3–9.0mmol of glucose per litre of blood has to be maintained. If too much glucose is present in the bloodstream insulin is released so that the excess can be converted into liver and muscle glycogen. Should the blood glucose level fall the liver glycogen can be converted back to glucose by the hormones adrenaline and glucagon. Muscle glycogen however is not converted back into glucose but is used up in muscle activity. Surplus blood glucose can also be converted to fats and stored in adipose tissue.

The accumulation of glucose in the blood is termed hyperglycaemia.

■ Symptoms and causes of diabetes mellitus

Diabetes may be hereditary, and although it can develop at any age, 80% of cases occur after the age of 50. It is slightly commoner in young males than young females but middle-aged women are more often affected than men of the same age-group. There is an association between obesity and diabetes and it may be precipitated by stress or infection. Diabetes may also develop as a secondary feature to another disorder, e.g. abnormal levels of other hormones in the blood (growth hormone, thyroxine, adrenaline), disease of the pancreas (pancreatitis, carcinoma). Diabetes may also develop following the administration of certain drugs (corticosteroids).

The manifestations of diabetes vary considerably, and the disorder when it develops in older people may be very gradual in onset, indeed glucosuria may be found during a routine medical examination. Some of the patients in the older age-group may present with the complications of diabetes, e.g. peripheral vascular disease, numbness or pains in the limbs, infections, or impaired sight. Some older women may seek the doctor's advice because of troublesome pruritus in the vulval region.

Other patients may present with classical symptoms of diabetes including loss of weight due to the mobilization of fat and the breakdown of protein; tiredness because there is insufficient glucose available to produce heat and energy; an increased urinary output because the glycosuria causes an osmotic diuresis and as a consequence the patient is drinking larger quantities (polydypsia). This may lead to dehydration and an electrolyte imbalance.

Other patients may present as medical emergencies when a precipitating factor may or may not be obvious. It is the accumulation of ketone bodies in the blood which may cause the patient to go into a coma (hyperglycaemic or diabetic coma). Fats can only be effectively metabolized while carbohydrate metabolism is proceeding normally. Due to the inefficient carbohydrate metabolism in diabetes, fats are not properly metabolized and an accumulation of ketone bodies develops. This is toxic to the brain if the accumulation rises beyond a certain level in the blood. This type of onset is sudden and severe and is more common in the younger age-groups.

■ Investigations

The investigations performed include:
a Testing the urine for glucose and ketone bodies.
b 24-hour urine collection for estimation of glucose present.
c Random blood sugar tests.
d Glucose tolerance test (oral).

■ Management of the patient with diabetes

The treatment involves active participation by the patient so that he fully understands the situation and everything that it is going to involve, as eventually he will be managing himself. The success of treatment is largely dependent on the patient. The exact treatment depends on the severity of the diabetes but a dietary regime is always necessary. The diabetes may be controlled by diet alone, or the combination of diet and hypoglycaemic drugs, or diet and insulin. All patients are treated individually and individual regimes may have to be changed over the course of time.

Education of the patient in relation to the disease, though time consuming, is of paramount importance. Urine testing, blood testing, the administration and dosage of insulin, knowledge of certain drugs and circumstances which may aggravate the diabetes, e.g. exercise, illness, and stress, should be thoroughly explained. If stabilization can take place at home under close supervision or in the hospital outpatient department while the patient is maintaining his usual activities in an environment that he knows, all the better. If this is not possible then hospitalization is necessary.

The aim of treatment is to correct the hyperglycaemia and glycosuria, maintain the appropriate body-weight and prevent the development of complications.

■ Diet

The dietary management of the diabetic patient is important and individual considerations have to be made for each patient, noting the patient's food habits, family and socio-economic background, sex, age, occupation and weight. When considering the total calorie intake all the above have to be taken into account. When the number of calories has been established these are then allocated between the carbohydrates, fats and proteins. The proportion of carbohydrates in terms of calories is usually less than that in the average diet, with an increase in the calories provided by the proteins, if this is possible. However, sufficient carbohydrates have to be given to ensure adequate fat metabolism thus preventing the development of ketonuria. The fat in the diet is regulated to meet the total calorie requirement.

Many methods are used in the calculation of diets for the diabetic and an exchange system has been devised to allow variety in the diet and to prevent the monotony which may develop if the patient had to adhere to the same diet sheet. It is important that the patient fully understands the exchange system, and if other members of the family are involved in the preparation of food it should also be explained to them. Accurate measurement of portions of food may also be necessary, particularly at the outset, and if the diabetes is controlled by insulin or hypoglycaemic agents. It may not be necessary for patients to abstain from taking alcohol but they must be aware of the calorific and/or carbohydrate content, and to consume it in moderation.

■ Treatment by insulin

Insulin is a protein and cannot, therefore, be given orally as it would be destroyed by the gastric juices. It is prepared from the pancreas of cattle and sheep so that it may be given parenterally. Diabetics who are not usually controlled by insulin may require it in some circumstances such as surgery, pregnancy or illness. Most of the patients requiring insulin therapy for their diabetes are children and young adults. The risks of hypoglycaemia should be borne in mind when a patient is receiving insulin.

There are different types of insulin which vary in the speed of effect and the length of time for which they are effective. Often combinations of insulins are used to suit individual patients (for more detail on the types and effects of insulin the student should refer to more comprehensive texts). The nurse must be familiar with the types of insulin used, as well as the various strengths and syringes that may be used specifically for the administration of insulin. The physician's advice should always be sought regarding the mixing of insulins. The insulin should be correctly stored and expiry dates noted. The sites used for injection include arm, thigh and abdomen, and should be rotated. Urine tests and blood sugar estimations are monitored while the patient is being stabilized, and the patient is taught to test his own urine and/or blood. The possible side-effects of insulin include hypoglycaemia and insulin resistance (rare). A patient may be allowed to experience a hypoglycaemic state under supervision so that he recognizes the early symptoms. He can be advised to carry glucose tablets or sugar lumps with him for emergencies. Manifestations of hypoglycaemia are as a result of the low blood sugar and its effects on the central nervous system and may lead to a (hypoglycaemic or insulin) coma. Treatment is aimed at raising the blood glucose level.

■ **Oral hypoglycaemic agents**

These drugs lower the blood glucose level by either augmenting insulin secretion (sulphonylureas) or increasing uptake of glucose (biguanides). The risk of hypoglycaemia is reduced with these drugs but does still exist with sulphonylureas and the patient must still be aware of the possibilities. Like the patient receiving insulin he must pay attention to diet and changes in day-to-day routine activities.

■ **General care**

The patient must be fully aware of the care that he must take of himself as far as general hygiene measures are concerned, the importance of avoiding infection as far as possible, adjusting the diet to suit energy expenditure, the importance of urine testing and management of insulin administration or hypoglycaemic agents.

The patient must carry a diabetic identification card containing appropriate information and he should appreciate that he will always be under the supervision of a physician and have to attend the outpatient department at regular intervals, although the interval will increase in length as he becomes better able to cope with his condition.

■ **Diabetic keto-acidosis**

There are degrees of diabetic crisis, therefore a state of coma need not exist before a medical emergency situation is present. Diabetic keto-acidosis is a serious complication of uncontrolled diabetes in which there is an accumulation of glucose in the blood as well as subsequent accumulation of ketone bodies, eventually giving rise to acidosis. The glycosuria causes an osmotic disturbance in the electrolyte balance.

Factors which may precipitate a diabetic crisis include infection, gastrointestinal disturbances, omission of insulin, alteration of dietary intake and undiagnosed diabetes mellitus. Diabetic acidosis develops gradually over several days, the patient experiencing thirst, polyuria, glycosuria, tiredness and weakness, nausea, vomiting, shallow rapid respirations, dryness of the mouth and skin, and the pulse may be weak and rapid with hypotension. Unless the patient receives prompt medical attention he will become comatosed.

□ *Treatment*
The aim of treatment in diabetic crisis is to:
a reduce the blood glucose level by stimulating its utilization by the body cells and prevent the accumulation of ketone bodies;
b correct the dehydration and electrolyte imbalance and treat the precipitating cause, e.g. infection.

Soluble insulin is usually given by the intravenous and intramuscular routes, e.g. Actrapid 6 units hourly until the blood pH is less than 7.3; if necessary the blood glucose level is maintained by intravenous glucose. Fluid replacement is by intravenous therapy. The fluids prescribed depend on the degree of acidosis and throughout the course of treatment regular laboratory estimations are made of the blood glucose levels, plasma bicarbonate and potassium, and urea. Following the administration of insulin, potassium as well as glucose will move from the extracellular fluid into the cell and potassium supplements in the infusion may be considered necessary. Antibiotic therapy is commenced and the patient catheterized so that the urine output can be monitored. Blood glucose is measured hourly. An electrocardiogram may also be performed to detect any changes in the heart's activity due to hypokalaemia and frequent regular observations are made of the respiratory and pulse rates and blood pressure. If the patient is vomiting a nasogastric tube may be passed and if the patient is in a coma measures should be taken to maintain a clear airway.

■ PRACTICE QUESTIONS

1 *What do you understand by the following terms?*
   a Thyroxine.
   b Goitre.
   c Toxic goitre.
   d Thyrotoxicosis.
   e Euthyroid.
   f Myxoedema.

   g Parathormone.

   h Thyrocalcitonin.

   i Exophthalmos.

   j Basal metabolic rate.

   k Carbimazole.

   l Islets of Langerhans.

   m Insulin.

   n Glucose tolerance test.

   o Osmotic diuresis.

   p Diabetic coma.

   q Insulin coma.

   r Oral hypoglycaemic agents.

   s Thyrotoxic heart disease.

   t Cretinism.

2 *Briefly explain the following:*

   a The accumulation of ketone bodies which occurs in uncontrolled diabetes mellitus.

   b The importance of taking food following the administration of insulin when diabetes is controlled by insulin injections.

   c Why glucose appears in the urine in diabetes mellitus.

   d Why the sites used for insulin injections should be rotated.

   e The reasons for hypoglycaemia.

   f Why is it particularly important to care for the skin and feet of the diabetic patient?

   g Why a patient on insulin is always advised to carry sugar lumps or glucose tablets with him.

   h The reasons for a patient with thyrotoxicosis feeling uneasy in an environment that is warm or feeling unduly hot and sweaty in an environment which most people would consider to be comfortable.

   i Why the blood cholesterol levels are estimated as a means of assessing thyroid activity.

   j Why radioactive iodine is effective in the treatment of thyrotoxicosis.

3 *Mark the following statements true or false:*

   a An endemic goitre may develop in those areas where there is inadequate iodine in the natural resources.

   b A semi-fluid substance is deposited under the skin of patients with myxoedema.

   c Thyrocalcitonin increases the blood calcium level.

   d Tetany is caused by an increase in the concentration of parathormone in the blood.

   e Thyroxine increases the blood glucose level by promoting the formation of glucose from amino acids.

f Insulin is given subcutaneously as it would be destroyed in the gastro-intestinal tract.

g Insulin zinc suspension lente acts quickly and has a short-term effect on lowering the blood sugar level.

h A constant and adequate supply of glucose is necessary for normal brain activity.

i The early signs and symptoms of hypoglycaemia include hunger, weakness and dehydration.

j In the state of hypoglycaemia the patient's urine contains no sugar.

k Patients with diabetes are more prone to develop conditions affecting the circulatory system.

l The release of insulin is stimulated by a low blood sugar level.

m Ketosis comes on more quickly than hypoglycaemia.

n Liver glycogen can be made from surplus amino acids and fats as well as from carbohydrate sources.

■ **Answers**

1 *a* Hormone produced by the thyroid gland from iodine and protein.

   b Enlargement of the thyroid gland.

   c Goitre associated with hyperactivity and oversecretion of thyroid hormone.

   d Clinical state produced due to oversecretion of thyroid hormone.

   e State of normal thyroid activity.

   f Clinical state produced due to underactivity of thyroid hormone.

   g Hormone secreted by the parathyroid glands.

   h Hormone produced by thyroid gland which lowers the plasma calcium levels.

   i Protrusion of the eyeballs.

   j A measurement of the oxygen requirements of the body when at rest.

   k An antithyroid drug. It interferes with the formation of thyroxine.

   l Groups of cells scattered throughout the pancreas which carry out the endocrine functions of the gland.

   m Hormone produced by the beta cells of the islets of Langerhans.

   n A diagnostic test used to determine the patient's tolerance of glucose.

   o The presence of substances in the glomerular filtrate usually absorbed by the renal tubules causes an increase in the urinary output, e.g. glucose, due to the osmotic pressure they exert.

   p A coma which develops as a result of the accumulation of ketone bodies and a high blood sugar level.

   q A coma which may occur as a result of a low blood sugar level when the brain is deprived of glucose.

   r Drugs that may be taken orally to lower the blood sugar levels.

    s Changes in the heart's action as a result of the increase in the circulating thyroxine.

    t A condition caused by deficiency of thyroxine in infancy and childhood.

2 *a* In uncontrolled diabetes the metabolism of carbohydrates is inadequate, and unless carbohydrates are metabolized normally the fats will not be adequately metabolized, with the subsequent development of ketone bodies which accumulate in the body.

    b The administration of insulin will cause a fall in the blood sugar levels and if the patient fails to take a meal a state of hypoglycaemia develops.

    c If the body is producing insufficient quantities of insulin, glucose will accumulate in the blood. When the amount of glucose present is sufficient to exceed the renal threshold, glucose will appear in the urine.

    d Frequent use of the same site causes fibrosing and scarring of the tissues which will delay the rate of absorption of insulin.

    e Delaying or omitting a meal following the administration of insulin; miscalculation resulting in overdose of insulin; exercising more than usual; vomiting or diarrhoea due to gastro-intestinal upsets.

    f There appears to be an increased incidence of degenerative vascular changes in the diabetic patient, giving rise to defective circulation and these changes in the lower limbs often lead to gangrene. Prevention of injury to skin is important, as well as advice about well fitting shoes and visits to the chiropodist for foot care.

    g The patient receiving insulin should be aware that under certain circumstances the blood sugar levels may fall below normal giving rise to the state of hypoglycaemia. Taking sugar in a concentrated form will help alleviate the symptoms, following which the patient should rest for a few hours.

    h Excess thyroxine increases the metabolic rate with a subsequent increase in the heat produced, giving rise to skin which is hot and sweaty.

    i Myxoedema is associated with a high blood cholesterol level, thyrotoxicosis with a low level. Thyroxine increases the excretion of cholesterol in bile.

    j The thyroid tissue is destroyed by radio-activity, reducing the formation of thyroxine.

3 *a* True   *e* True   *i* False   *m* False
    b True   *f* True   *j* True   *n* True
    c False   *g* False   *k* True
    d False   *h* True   *l* False

8 The stomach and the small and large intestines

The purpose of this chapter is to:
1 State the structure and function of the stomach and intestines.
2 Describe the common diseases and investigations that may be required.
3 Describe the total management and nursing care of patients with diseases affecting the stomach and intestines.

The structures of the stomach, small intestine and large intestine are similar in that they have four layers. From the outside in they are the peritoneum, the muscle coat, the submucous coat and the mucous membrane. The variations that occur are due to the functions of each portion.

The stomach is the widest portion of these tubular structures. The mucous membrane of the stomach consists of irregular longitudinal ridges (rugae). The tubular glands consist of different kinds of cells which secrete mucus, hydrochloric acid and a fluid containing enzymes. The muscular coat consists of an oblique layer of smooth muscle, as well as the usual circular and longitudinal layers. The enzyme pepsin is produced in the stomach (secreted as pepsinogen) and acts on proteins, breaking them down into proteoses and peptones. The stimulation of gastric juice is under nervous and hormonal control. The hormone responsible is gastrin which is released as a result of nervous stimulation and the presence of food in the stomach. When fat is present in the food another hormone, enterogastrone, is produced by the stomach and small intestine, which slows down the movements of the stomach and delays emptying. The function of the stomach is to store and churn food, breaking it down into smaller particles, mixing it with gastric juice and, over a period of 3–4 hours, it is passed on in small quantities to the duodenum as chyme. The stomach also produces the intrinsic factor. Apart from water and alcohol very little absorption takes place in the stomach.

The left gastric artery, the splenic artery and the hepatic artery supply the stomach with blood.

The small intestine is continuous with the stomach at one end and the large intestine at the other. It consists of the duodenum, the jejunum and the ileum. The functions of the small intestine are to continue with the digestion of food, its absorption, and also to move the chyme along by means of peristalsis. The mucous membrane is designed to facilitate the process of absorption by the presence of villi on its surface. These are

Summary of juices in the small intestine, their stimulation, the enzymes present, and their action.

Juice	Stimulated by	Enzymes present	Action
Pancreatic juice	Nervous control (Vagal stimulation)	Pancreatic amylase	Splits starch and dextrins to maltose
	Hormones (Secretin Pancreozymin)	Lipase	Hydrolyses neutral fats and fatty acids
		Precursors—trypsinogen activated to trypsin by enterokinase, chymotrypsinogen activated to chymotrypsin by trypsin	Breaks down proteins to polypeptides
Intestinal juice	Mechanical stimulation of intestinal wall	Maltase ⎫ Sucrase ⎬ Lactase ⎭	Converts disaccharides into monosaccharides
		Erepsin	Converts polypeptides into amino acids
		Enterokinase	Converts trypsinogen into active trypsin
Bile	Hormone cholecystokinin	(Bile salts)	Increases activity of pancreatic lipase, emulsifies fats

covered by columnar epithelium and scattered among them are goblet cells which secrete mucus. Each villus is fed by a capillary plexus and contains a blind-ended lymph capillary called a lacteal. Intestinal juice is produced by cells lining the crypts of Lieberkuhn. Large lymph nodules are found in the ileum called Peyer's patches. An alkaline secretion is produced by Brunner's glands in the submucous coat of the duodenum to protect the mucosa from the acid and enzymes from the stomach.

In addition to the intestinal juice produced, pancreatic juice and bile also enter the small intestine (duodenum) at the ampulla of Vater. These secretions are all alkaline and help to neutralize the acid content of chyme.

When digested food has been sufficiently broken down it is absorbed in the small intestine. Water and digested products (including some fat) are absorbed into the bloodstream and carried by the hepatic portal system to the liver. About two-thirds of the digested fat passes to the lacteals in the villi and is carried by the lymph vessels as chyle. It is then emptied into the veins at the root of the neck via the thoracic duct.

Blood is supplied to the small intestine via the superior mesenteric artery.

The large intestine consists of the caecum, appendix, ascending, transverse and descending colon, pelvic colon, rectum and anal canal. The large intestine is shorter in length than the small intestine but has a larger lumen. The ileum is continuous with the caecum and the orifice is guarded by the ileocaecal valve. The longitudinal muscle fibres in the muscular coat are incomplete therefore giving the intestine a sacculated appearance caused by the bulging of the circular muscle fibres. The mucous membrane consists of columnar epithelium, goblet cells which secrete mucus, but no villi are present. The functions of the large intestine include the absorption of water, lubrication for the passage of faeces and storage of faeces in the distal colon. The presence of bacteria synthesizes vitamins K and B.

When food enters the stomach it gives rise to the gastro-colic reflex, causing a rush of peristalsis through the large intestine, moving its contents on to the rectum. The desire to defaecate is brought about by the subsequent distension of the rectum. The anal canal is guarded by two sphincters, the internal sphincter composed of smooth muscle under the control of the autonomic nervous system, and the external sphincter composed of striated muscle under voluntary control (except for the first few years of life). The higher centres control the external sphincter and defaecation will only take place when this sphincter is relaxed. Defaecation is aided by contraction of the abdominal muscles and diaphragm which increases the intra-abdominal pressure.

The blood supply to the appendix, caecum, ascending colon and the proximal two-thirds of the colon is via the superior mesenteric artery. The remaining distal third of the transverse colon, descending and pelvic colon and rectum is supplied by the inferior mesenteric artery. Veins draining blood from the stomach and small intestines pour their blood into tributaries, which empty into the portal vein to the liver. The food materials contained in the blood are then metabolized by the liver cells. This system is called the hepatic portal system.

■ SPECIFIC INVESTIGATIONS WHICH MAY BE CARRIED OUT ON THE STOMACH AND INTESTINES

■ Endoscopic procedures

These procedures involve passing an instrument to which a light is attached, into an organ so that it can be visually examined. Some tubes have special glass fibres in them which transmit light on to the mucosa and cameras may also be attached to the instrument so that pictures may be taken. An endoscope may be used to view the oesophagus (oesophagoscopy), the stomach (gastroscopy), the sigmoid colon, rectum and anal canal (sigmoidoscopy). The rectum and anal canal can be directly viewed by means of a proctoscope. A biopsy may be performed by means of an endoscope. Prior to an endoscope being passed into the oesophagus or stomach the patient will have to refrain from eating and drinking for 6–8 hours, and also sign a consent form. The patient may or may not require a general anaesthetic. A local anaesthetic is usually administered for the back of the throat, either as lozenges or a spray. A sedative may be given, dentures and jewellery removed and a gown placed on the patient. The bladder is emptied before the patient leaves the ward to go to the theatre. On return fluids and food are withheld for 4–6 hours so that time is given for the effect of the local anaesthetic to wear off.

The preparation for sigmoidoscopy and proctoscopy include preparation of the bowel by the administration of an enema, and a low residue diet may be taken on the day prior to the examination. This procedure is often carried out in the ward.

■ **Special radiological examinations**

The oesophagus, stomach and intestines can be outlined by giving the patient a radio-opaque substance (barium sulphate) to take orally (barium swallow or barium meal) prior to the radiological examination. The patient is advised not to eat anything after the last meal the evening before the examination. On completion of the gastro-intestinal series the radiologist will notify the nurses regarding the commencement of diet for the patient. As barium is a chalky substance a mouthwash may be given when the patient returns to the ward. An aperient may have to be administered the following day as barium may cause constipation.

The preparations for a barium enema for examination of the large intestine and rectum include withholding food for up to 24 hours prior to the procedure (fluids are allowed), and preparation of the bowel by the administration of an evacuant enema. Specific instructions regarding the preparation are usually received from the department. A mild aperient may be required to prevent constipation from developing due to residual barium.

■ **Gastric analysis tests**

These may be performed to estimate the contents of the stomach at a given time. Gastric contents may be examined for the presence of bile, blood, organisms, the concentration of hydrochloric acid and to estimate the amount of gastric secretions produced. A tubeless gastric analysis test is also possible by first fasting the patient and then administering a gastric stimulant and a substance containing a dye combined with a resin and water. If hydrochloric acid is produced in response to the stimulant, the acid will free the dye from the resin and the former will be absorbed and excreted in urine. The patient provides a urine specimen two hours after the drugs are given and the amount of dye present is measured. The concentration of the dye is an indication of the amount of acid released.

■ Examination of stools

It may be necessary to obtain specimens of stool for analysis. Due to diseases of the gastro-intestinal tract, blood, parasites and excessive fats may be present in the faeces, as well as specific organisms. Containers specifically for stool specimens are usually available and these reduce the handling of stools to a minimum. The patient should be told that specimens are required so that he informs the nursing staff when stools have been passed into the appropriate receptacle which will have been provided. If any abnormalities are seen with the naked eye a specimen should be retained for inspection by the doctor.

■ COMMON CONDITIONS OF THE GASTRO-INTESTINAL TRACT

■ Peptic ulceration

This is the term used to describe the erosion of the mucosa of the lower end of the oesophagus, the stomach and duodenum, due to the digestive action of pepsin and hydrochloric acid.

Why some people develop peptic ulcers is not yet known but possible causes are the inability of the mucosa to provide sufficient resistance to the hydrochloric acid and pepsin produced, malnutrition and poor blood supply, and hormonal factors. Predisposing factors include a strong family history of peptic ulceration, stress, excessive alcohol consumption and smoking. It has also been found that there is an association between peptic ulceration and blood group O and that a seasonal variation in the recurrence of symptoms exists.

☐ *Signs and symptoms*
The history, as related by the patient, frequently extends over a number of months or possibly years. However, the patient may present as a surgical emergency following perforation of the ulcer, or following haemorrhage due to the erosion of a blood vessel at the site of the ulcer. Patients often complain of pain or discomfort and the site referred to varies from person

to person. The positive pointing sign is said to be present when the patient can point with one finger or a group of fingers when asked to locate the site of pain. The pain may be felt in the epigastric region, over the ribs or in the back. The pain may also be related to meals and vomiting.

Dyspepsia is usually present and the patient may also complain of heartburn. As well as taking a medical history the doctor may also ask for some or all of the following investigations:

1 A full blood count
2 A specimen of stool for occult blood
3 A barium meal
4 Gastric analysis
5 Endoscopic examination.

The treatment involves rest which may or may not be achieved in the home under the supervision of the general practitioner. If the home is not conducive to achieving the physical and mental rest required, then hospitalization is necessary. Sedatives may also be prescribed for those patients who are particularly anxious.

The type of diet prescribed for the patient is determined by the physician, the severity of the symptoms, and the patient's response to a dietary regime. A modified milk diet may be prescribed, or a fairly liberal diet where the patient avoids foods known to irritate his condition. Patients are advised to eat smaller but more frequent meals or possibly eat between meals to avoid the feeling of hunger. Patients are usually advised to avoid chemically irritating foods, gravies, tea and coffee because of their caffeine content, and alcohol. It may be that during the acute stage a continuous intragastric milk drip may be prescribed.

Drug therapy may include antacids for the relief of pain. Some antacids cause diarrhoea, others constipation, a combination of varied antacids will help to prevent these side-effects. Reduction of gastric secretion and motility may be achieved by the administration of a synthetic anti-cholinergic drug, e.g. propantheline.

Drugs of a liquorice derivative may also be prescribed due to their healing properties, e.g. Caved-S.

Patients are also advised to refrain from smoking.

When medical treatment fails to heal the ulcer and symptoms persist, surgery may have to be considered. (See *Surgical Nursing* in this series.)

■ **Acute gastro-enteritis**

This is a term used to describe inflammation of the mucosa of the stomach and small intestine due to food poisoning which develops up to 48 hours after taking contaminated food or fluids. The food poisoning may be caused by the exotoxins produced by some organisms, e.g. staphylococcus, pyogenes and possibly haemolytic and non-haemolytic streptococcus, and the salmonella group. Outbreaks of food poisoning occur more frequently in institutions where large amounts of food are prepared. Left-over food may be kept for re-use, and the storage of such food under inadequate conditions is an important factor in the causation of such a disease, due to multiplication of organisms in the food while it is being stored.

Gastro-enteritis is usually found to affect other members of the family, or other members of a group of people within an institution, and is in itself suggestive of food poisoning. The usual signs and symptoms consist of nausea, vomiting, abdominal pain and diarrhoea and the severity of the symptoms depends on the amount ingested and the causative poison. The duration of onset of symptoms may be indicative of whether the poison is chemical, exotoxic or bacterial, the latter often developing within 12–48 hours of ingestion. The former are usually much more rapid in onset.

If the patient is admitted to hospital a specimen of stool and vomit may be obtained and sent to the laboratory for bacteriological examination. The treatment depends on the severity of the symptoms; rest and oral fluids may be all that is required. A stomach washout may be necessary in some instances and appropriate antidotes prescribed. Fluid and electrolyte balance may have to be restored by the administration of intravenous fluids. As the patient responds to treatment a light diet may be gradually introduced. Drugs which may be prescribed include, for example, kaolin to control the diarrhoea, and possibly an antibiotic.

■ The malabsorption syndrome

This term is used to cover those disorders associated with a defect which prevents the absorption of certain foodstuffs, giving rise to signs and symptoms which occur as a result of malabsorption. Absorption may be affected due to atrophy of the villi, the presence of bacteria in the small bowel, a decrease in the surface area of the bowel, a deficiency of enzymes so that foodstuffs are inadequately broken down for absorption, and there may be a disease present which affects the flow of lymph or blood to the intestine. Distension of the abdomen is usually present. The diarrhoea in such cases usually contains a large amount of fats. Deficiency of vitamin K may give rise to a tendency to haemorrhage. Anaemia may also be present as other vitamins necessary for red blood cell formation are inadequately absorbed. Tetany may occur due to calcium deficiency. Signs of nutritional deficiency may be noted, e.g. rickets, soreness of tongue, stomatitis and changes in the hair and nails. The doctor may order a barium meal and follow-through studies, a biopsy of the intestinal mucosa and absorption tests, which include collection of stools over a period of 3–5 days for analysis of their fat content. Blood will also be obtained for a full blood count and haemoglobin concentration, prothrombin and serum calcium levels. Tests may also be necessary to establish the presence of pancreatic disease.

The *treatment* of malabsorption syndrome includes replacement of all the nutritional deficiencies by the administration of the appropriate substances. These may include calcium gluconate and vitamins D, K and B. Iron and folic acid may be given orally or parenterally depending on the severity of anaemia, and vitamin B_{12} deficiency is treated by the administration of hydroxocobalamin. Oedema may require the administration of diuretics and protein may be replaced in the diet. If the patient's condition is severe, intravenous fluid therapy may be necessary to correct any dehydration and deficiency of electrolytes. If the cause of the syndrome cannot be found the patient may respond to a gluten-free diet.

■ Crohn's disease (regional ileitis)

The symptoms of this disease usually begin in the twenties to thirties age-group and its cause is unknown. As the term regional ileitis suggests there are localized patches of non-specific inflammation which may become ulcerated, oedematous and infected in the lower end of the ileum and sometimes the colon. The patient experiences periods of exacerbations and remissions and the history usually extends over a number of years. The patient may complain of colicky abdominal pain, associated with mild diarrhoea and loss of weight. A fixed mass which is tender may also be present in the right iliac fossa. Anaemia and a low grade fever may also be present. A barium follow-through examination is an important aid to diagnosis. Microscopic examination of the faeces may be useful. A Mantoux test may be done to exclude tuberculosis of the ileo-caecal region.

During an acute exacerbation, rest is prescribed with a high protein low residue diet and vitamin supplements. A short course of sulphasalazine may be ordered, or alternatively an antibiotic to combat secondary infection. Corticosteroid therapy may also be prescribed during an acute phase. Surgical treatment of the disease may also be considered, although this is not usually carried out during an acute phase of the disease. (See *Surgical Nursing*.)

■ Ulcerative colitis

This is the term used for inflammation and ulceration of the colon, and because no specific organism has been found to cause these changes it is often referred to as non-specific ulcerative colitis. The disease process usually begins in the rectum and spreads to the colon. Diseases, involving the joints and skin, accompanying ulcerative colitis have given rise to the consideration of its being an auto-immune disease. It has also been noted that patients with ulcerative colitis are emotionally immature, extremely 'fussy' tidy people and that acute exacerbations often occur following an emotional crisis. Whether the psychological make-up of the patient is a contributory factor or develops as a result of the disease is not clear. The disease usually begins in early adult life and varies in severity as does the extent of the colonic involvement. It is serious and chronic in that recovery is rare although long periods of remission may be experienced. Diarrhoea with blood and mucus is a feature of the disease accompanied by abdominal pain, loss of weight, anaemia, pyrexia and changes in skin as a result of vitamin deficiency.

□ *Investigations*
These may include:
Blood examination; full blood count; erythrocyte sedimentation rate (ESR) and electrolyte estimation
Proctoscopy; sigmoidoscopy
Barium enema
Stools for microscopy.

□ *Treatment*
The treatment depends on the severity of the disease. When the patient is admitted to hospital during an acute exacerbation complete bed rest is usually prescribed. Diet usually consists of high protein and calorie and low residue foods and avoiding all foods which may stimulate bowel activity, including fruits, very hot or very cold liquids. Vitamin supplements are also given if the patient is severely ill on admission. Foods and fluids may be withheld orally to reduce the activity of the intestines and intravenous therapy commenced. Drug therapy may include iron therapy for the anaemia and sulphasalazine has been shown to bring about remission. Corticosteroids may be prescribed for oral administration as well as corticosteroid enemas. Codeine phosphate may also be prescribed to control the diarrhoea and relieve abdominal pain. Surgical intervention may be considered necessary.

■ **Constipation and diarrhoea**

The pattern of emptying the bowels varies from one person to another, some may have a bowel action twice a day, others every two or three days, and both these patterns may be natural and healthy. Many people believe it is normal and healthy to have a bowel action daily and adopt a ritual of taking laxatives in order to achieve this, a natural rhythm is, therefore, never acquired.

□ *Constipation*

This term is used to describe a delay in the evacuation of faeces. It may develop due to local causes in the intestine, e.g. adhesions, megacolon, tumours, and haemorrhoids and anal fissure which cause pain on defaecation. Dehydration, depressive states and hypothyroidism may also give rise to constipation. The most common type of constipation is habit constipation or dyschezia when a person persistently fails to empty the bowels. Failure to empty the rectum may also be due to lack of roughage in the diet and in the elderly it may be due to muscle weakness of the abdomen and pelvic floor.

If an organic cause is found it is treated. Mild aperients may be prescribed for a patient who is feverish, to prevent the development of constipation. It is, however, important to establish with the patient his usual bowel habits. If constipation has developed, suppositories or a small enema may be given. For 'habit constipation', educating the patient about the importance of responding to the call to stool and re-training of bowel habits may be necessary, as well as taking an adequate diet and exercise to improve muscle tone. An important complication of constipation particularly in the elderly is faecal impaction which may cause partial or complete obstruction.

□ *Diarrhoea*

This is the term used to describe the passage of unformed stools. Diarrhoea can be acute or chronic. Acute diarrhoea occurs as a result of infected food and chemical poisonings, alcohol, and dietetic indiscretions. Chronic diarrhoea may be due to lesions of the small or large intestine following gastric surgery and vagotomy, thyrotoxicosis and nervous diarrhoea.

To establish the cause of the diarrhoea the faeces require examination, a barium meal, barium enema, or endoscopy may be indicated.

■ SUMMARY OF THE NURSING CARE OF PATIENTS WITH GASTRO-INTESTINAL DISEASES

■ Position in the ward

A patient with gastro-enteritis may require isolation and a side-room should be made available. Patients whose symptoms include diarrhoea, where frequent visits to the toilet are necessary, should be placed near a toilet provided they are allowed up. If complete bed rest is prescribed it may be less embarrassing for the patient, while the diarrhoea remains, to have a side-room with its greater degree of privacy. A patient with a peptic ulcer may benefit from the quiet and rest afforded by a single room.

■ Position in bed

Immobilization is usually determined by the patient. However, movement in bed must be encouraged, particularly patients who are afraid of stimulating another bowel movement. The implications of not moving should be explained to the patient and limb exercises to prevent joint contractures should also be employed at regular intervals. A patient with acute diarrhoea may benefit from lying flat as this may help to reduce peristaltic activity.

■ Skin and general hygiene

The patient's ability to care for his own general hygiene should be carefully assessed and assistance given accordingly. The nursing care should be planned so that the patient receives adequate rest periods. Due to the possible nutritional deficiencies associated with malabsorption syndrome, Crohn's disease and ulcerative colitis, care must be taken to ensure that the skin remains intact. Washing and drying should be gentle, there should be frequent inspection of the skin, the patient should be moved and lifted clear of bedpans and the nurse should select appropriate aids to prevent the development of pressure sores. Particular attention should be paid to the skin in the anal region if diarrhoea is present, washing and drying and the application of a protective cream following each defaecation. The doctor may prescribe an ointment to be applied to the anus, if tenesmus is troublesome. Frequent change of linen may be required if the patient is pyrexial. Attention must also be paid to the hair and nails if the patient is unable to do this himself. The mouth should be kept clean at all times and facilities provided for the patient to maintain oral care. Extra mouthwashes may be required following a barium meal because much of the chalky material tends to collect and causes dryness of the mouth; also if the patient is vomiting or regurgitating, or is not eating or drinking. The nurse should observe the mouth for changes which may occur as a result of nutritional deficiencies – soreness, ulceration, or signs of gastro-intestinal disturbances such as a coated tongue or halitosis.

■ Eating and drinking

Specific reference to the importance of diets in gastro-intestinal disease has already been made, however, the nurse must be familiar with the types of diet prescribed for individual patients and to observe that the patient is taking the diet. Patients may require some explanation as to when certain foods have to be avoided and why others are necessary. Diet is often such an important part of treatment that great skill is required to convince the reluctant patient. Some foods have to be avoided altogether: the patient on a gluten-free diet, for example, requires information on how and where to obtain gluten-free foods and flour. Other patients, for example those with ulcerative colitis, may find that as soon as they begin a meal they require a bedpan; in such a case the food should be removed and kept warm even though the patient may be reluctant to continue the meal afterwards. It is important that time is taken to talk to the patient with a peptic ulcer so that he understands the importance of taking meals that are regular and unhurried. Members of the family involved in the preparation of meals should also attend the discussions. Vitamins may also be prescribed to supplement the diet. The reasons for withholding food and drink prior to certain investigations should similarly be fully explained to the patient. When the patient is severely ill nutrition and hydration may be maintained by intravenous therapy. It is possible to obtain fluids which are high in nutritional value and these may be used to supplement the diet.

The patient's nutritional state may require close observation and the patient may be weighed daily, or less frequently if the patient becomes anxious about his weight. Note is made of any food which may increase the diarrhoea present.

■ Elimination

If a patient is admitted to hospital with acute diarrhoea, as in gastro-enteritis, strict precautions should be taken with the stools until tests have shown them not to be infected. Investigations involving the rectum, and the administration of suppositories and enemas can be a source of much embarrassment for the patient, so that time set aside to explain why these measures are necessary, and a well prepared environment free from interruptions, will help to maintain privacy and alleviate much of the anxiety felt by the patient. The patient's co-operation and confidence should be gained in relation to the collection of specimens, as in some instances all the stools passed for up to five days may have to be obtained for laboratory investigations. Containers for this purpose are usually supplied by the laboratory.

Patients with diarrhoea are usually anxious that they might soil the bed if they do not receive the bedpan in time; as far as possible this anxiety should be allayed and it may be necessary for a covered pan to be left near the bedside and replaced by a clean one as soon as it has been used. Facilities for handwashing must be made available to the patient after each use of the bedpan.

The possibility of constipation should be borne in mind when a patient is receiving antacids.

■ Observations

Observations of the temperature, pulse and blood pressure are carried out as frequently as is dictated by the condition of the patient. When the patient is receiving intravenous infusion therapy its maintenance is continuously observed, and the amount of fluid infused, urinary output and an estimation of diarrhoea, are recorded on a fluid balance chart. In some instances anaemia may be treated by blood transfusions and the usual specific observations are carried out at regular intervals unless more frequent intervals are indicated. Plasma infusions may also be prescribed and administered, to restore the continual loss of protein in the stools, e.g. in ulcerative colitis.

The patient's general condition is observed – the degree of weakness and tiredness, response to the illness, attitude and mood. Changes in behaviour around visiting times are noted and in some instances screening of visitors may be necessary.

Any vomit is observed for amount, colour and consistency, and if the patient is feeling nauseated a clean vomit bowl covered with a paper towel should be kept near at hand with adequate supplies of paper tissues.

■ Communication

Communication with the patient and his or her close relations is extremely important. The need for a patient with a peptic ulcer to avoid stress and anxiety should be understood by both patient and family.

It may be necessary to discuss the possibility of surgery and ileostomy with these cases and the doctor and patient will require a certain degree of privacy in which to discuss such matters. The patient may have numerous questions to ask regarding surgery.

Both the patient and his family, where appropriate, should have an understanding of the disease and the reasons for the therapeutic advice that is given, and understand the necessity of avoiding certain foods.

Patients with certain chronic diseases, e.g. ulcerative colitis, should be encouraged to live as normal a life as possible and remain in their occupation. Life should be organized in such a way that neither work nor recreation is taxing for the patient, so that he may avoid exhaustion. All patients when discharged from hospital are advised that if they are worried about any aspect of their illness to consult their doctor.

■ PRACTICE QUESTIONS

1 *What is meant by the following terms:*
 a Hormone.
 b Enzyme.
 c Intrinsic factor.
 d Lacteal.
 e Enterokinase.
 f Secretin.
 g Peristalsis.
 h Segmentation.
 i Hepatic portal system.
 j Sigmoidoscopy.
 k Flatulence.
 l Anti-cholinergic drug.
 m Exotoxins.
 n Malabsorption syndrome.
 o Tenesmus.
 p Gastro–colic reflex.
 q 'Habit' constipation.
 r Acute diarrhoea.
 s Ulcerative colitis.
 t Diverticulitis.
 u Haematemesis.
 v Melaena.

2 *Briefly explain the following:*
 a How may a patient with severe ulcerative colitis become oedematous?
 b Why may anti-cholinergic drugs be prescribed for patients with peptic ulcers?
 c Why is a gluten-free diet prescribed for patients with coeliac disease?
 d Pain described as colic.
 e The possible complications of Crohn's disease.
 f Why perforation of a peptic ulcer is considered to be a dangerous complication.

3 *Mark the following statements true or false:*
 a Gastrin inhibits the secretion of gastric juice.
 b Sounds that are made by movement of fluid and gas in the intestines, which can be heard by the patient and others who may be close by, are called borborygmi.
 c Rennin is a substance produced in the stomach of some animals but not man.

    d Rigidity of the abdominal wall is never present in diseases of the gastro-intestinal tract.

    e Erepsin is an enzyme found in pancreatic juice.

    f Irritation of the phrenic nerve causes the diaphragm to go into spasm, giving rise to hiccoughs.

    g Anti-cholinergic drugs should not be given to patients with glaucoma or an enlarged prostate gland.

    h Megacolon is the term used to describe an excessively long colon.

    i Histamine and insulin both stimulate the secretion of gastric juice.

    j One of the possible complications of ulcerative colitis is perforation of an ulcerated portion of the bowel.

    k Chronic constipation may lead to the development of haemorrhoids.

■ Answers

1 *a* A chemical substance produced by endocrine glands which circulates in the blood to modify the action of distant organs.

    b A catalyst which brings about a chemical change. Enzymes are themselves proteins.

    c This is produced by the stomach and is necessary for the absorption of vitamin B_{12}.

    d Lymphatic vessels found in the small intestines.

    e An enzyme found in intestinal juice which is required for the conversion of trypsinogen into active trypsin.

    f A hormone which stimulates the production of pancreatic juice.

    g Waves of muscular activity in the intestine which serve to move the contents along the tube.

    h Muscular activity in the small intestine which serves to bring its contents into contact with the surface of the walls of the gut. This movement also helps to break up the food so that better contact with the digestive juices is achieved.

    i A system of veins which transport blood from the capillaries of the gastro-intestinal tract to the capillaries of the liver.

    j An endoscopic procedure used for visual examination of the rectum and sigmoid colon.

    k The presence of excessive amounts of gas in the gastro-intestinal tract.

    l Drugs which inhibit or interfere with the action of acetylcholine.

    m A toxin liberated by living bacteria into their environment.

    n Said to be present when there is failure to absorb essential foodstuffs from the alimentary tract.

    o Painful spasm of the anus.

p A wave of contraction of the colon accompanied by the desire to defaecate, as a result of food entering the stomach.

q Constipation which develops as a result of persistent failure to respond to the call to stool.

r Diarrhoea which results from dietary indiscretion, infection, food poisoning.

s Serious chronic disease where there are inflamed, ulcerated lesions present in the rectum and colon.

t Term used to describe inflammation of small pouches or sacs present in the wall of the intestine, thought to develop from weakness of the wall or increased pressure from within the intestine.

u The vomiting of blood.

v The passage of a black, tarry stool which contains blood from the gastro-intestinal tract.

2 *a* If proteins are lost to such an extent in the stools, oedema may develop if the liver cannot synthesize sufficient albumin to make good the loss.

b To reduce the motility and excess gastric secretions associated with patients who have peptic ulcers.

c Because patients with coeliac disease develop an intolerance to gluten which is a protein in wheat and rye.

d This is spasmodic in nature, arising from a hollow, muscular organ and usually due to obstruction in its lumen which may be partial or complete.

e Perforation, abscess formation, fistula and stenosis of the bowel.

f Gastric or duodenal contents will escape into the peritoneal cavity, giving rise to peritonitis. Urgent surgical intervention is required to close the perforation.

3 *a* False

b True

c False

d False

e False

f True

g True

h False

i True

j True

k True

Advice for examination preparation

Start your preparation well in advance of the examination. Make a realistic plan of action that you will be able to achieve.

1 Decide how many hours each day you can set aside for study/revision. 2 hours daily × 5 = 10 hours weekly.
2 Make a timetable and slot in all the subjects to be studied. The length of time you allocate depends on the level of difficulty.
3 Study in the same place each day. Sit at a desk or table and have the materials you need at hand, i.e. paper, pencils, crayons, textbooks, lecture notes and a rubber. Write in pencil so that mistakes or unwanted notes can be erased (paper is expensive).
4 You must work at concentrating on your task; don't allow yourself to think of anything else so that you waste time.
5 If you are tired or upset, relax before attempting to settle.
6 Work at each of the goals you have set yourself as widely as you can.
7 Reward yourself when a goal is achieved so that you associate pleasure with studying.
8 Success is not a matter of luck but of good planning and self-discipline.
9 Learning is an active process so:
   o Study using a logical approach. Sequence the material and go from each to more difficult concepts.
   o Don't try to learn chunks of material. Skim the passage and try to understand. Underline key words or sentences. Use a dictionary.
   o Overlearn material and consciously recall and reinforce your memory. Commit your thoughts to paper.
   o Use mnemonics as a memory aid.
   o Ask yourself questions, apply the material, compare with management of actual patients you have nursed. Have discussions with friends/tutors.
   o Ask your tutors for help if you do not understand the relevance of a topic.
   o Learn to draw and label line drawings correctly.
   o Test yourself using past examination questions.
   o Get your relatives or friends to ask questions.
10 Cultivate a fast reading style. Use several textbooks with your notes. Make your own notes when you have analysed the meaning of a passage. Begin to read with a question in mind and ask yourself

questions when you have read a paragraph/chapter. Read quickly then reread.

11 What you want to achieve is efficiency of study with economy of effort.

■ EXAMINATION TECHNIQUE

1 Listen to any instructions and follow them carefully. Be prepared with pens, pencils, a rubber and ruler.
2 Read the instructions on the examination paper and comply with them, i.e. start a question on a fresh page, number your questions carefully, write legibly. Note how many questions are to be attempted, how much time, is allowed, etc.
3 Essay questions test
   o Knowledge
   o Comprehension
   o Application
   o Communication
   o Synthesis.
4 Read carefully all the questions on both sides of the paper, identify all parts of each question.
   o Don't be concerned that others have started to write.
   o Select the questions you feel most able to answer.
   o Tick your selection in order of sequence.
   o Analyse the setting of the question. Is the scene in hospital or the community? What is the importance of age, sex, marital/social status, environment, psychological well-being, needs of the patient in the examiner's mind. Underline these points and develop them.
   o Note the essential points that have to be made in your answer in the margin of the paper.
   o Pay attention to the weighting of each part of the question, these should help you plan the time to be spent on each part.
   o Ten minutes spent in planning is the most effective way of using the examination time.
   o When you start to write:
      Answer the parts in order of *a, b, c, d*
      Write legibly, be logical (first things first)
      Concentrate on the main parts, don't waffle and repeat yourself
      If a diagram is asked for make a clear line drawing and label it clearly.
      Leave time at the end for reading your answers.

Remember that a good essay has an introduction, a development and a conclusion, and should be clear and concise. Remember also that each sentence requires a verb!

Further reading

Blackwell, C. C. and Weir, D. M. (1984). *Principles of Infection and Immunity in Patient Care*. Churchill Livingstone, Edinburgh.

Brunt, M. (1982). *Physiology in Nursing*. Harper and Row, London.

Faulkner, A. (1985). *Nursing – A Creative Approach*. Baillière Tindall, London.

Fream, W. C. (1985). *Notes on Medical Nursing*, 4th edition. Churchill Livingstone, Edinburgh.

Wilson, K. J. W. (1987). *Ross and Wilson Anatomy and Physiology in Health and Illness*, 6th edition. Churchill Livingstone, Edinburgh.

The *British National Formulary* (*BNF*) is published six-monthly by the British Medical Association and the Pharmaceutical Society of Great Britain. It is freely available in all hospitals.

Index